BIOCHEMISTRY RESEARCH TREN

Additional books in this series can be found on Nova's website under the Series tab.

Additional E-books in this series can be found on Nova's website under the E-books tab.

BIOCHEMISTRY RESEARCH TRENDS

URIC ACID

BIOLOGY, FUNCTIONS AND DISEASES

BIOCHEMISTRY RESEARCH TRENDS

URIC ACID

BIOLOGY, FUNCTIONS AND DISEASES

SANTIAGO E. CASTILLO
AND
ERNESTO W. MALDONADO
EDITORS

Nova Science Publishers, Inc.
New York

For permission to use material from this book please contact us:
Telephone 631-231-7269; Fax 631-231-8175
Web Site: http://www.novapublishers.com

Additional color graphics may be available in the e-book version of this book.

Library of Congress Cataloging-in-Publication Data

Uric acid : biology, functions, and diseases / editors, Santiago E. Castillo and Ernesto W. Maldonado.
p. ; cm.
Includes bibliographical references and index.
ISBN 978-1-62100-762-3 (hardcover)
I. Castillo, Santiago E. II. Maldonado, Ernesto W.
[DNLM: 1. Uric Acid. WJ 303]
612.4'61--dc23

2011039226

Published by Nova Science Publishers, Inc. † New York

Contents

Preface

Uric acid is the end-product of the purine metabolism in human beings. Most of this substance is in the form of monosodium urate in compartments with pH 7.4, such as plasma and extracellular fluids. In this book, the authors present current research in the study of the biology, functions and disease relating to uric acid. Topics discussed include the role of uric acid in the avian species; uric acid in multiple sclerosis and neurodegenerative diseases and the role of uric acid in metabolic syndrome and in hypertension and renal failure. (Imprint: Nova Biomedical).

Chapter I – Birds have a remarkable longevity for their body size despite an increased body temperature, higher metabolic rate, and increased blood glucose concentrations. Theoretically, birds should sustain a much higher degree of oxidative damage and processes leading to senescence such as glycoxidation of proteins and nucleic acids. Because this is not the case this suggests that birds have developed a more efficacious antioxidant defense system in order to cope with the oxidative burden. In actual fact birds have evolved into uric acid 'machines': uric acid is a potent antioxidant that is known to scavenge singlet oxygen, peroxy radicals, and hydroxyl radicals. Uric acid also binds with other primary radicals in addition to neutralizing iron ion complexes, which could signify additional antioxidant capabilities. Uric acid has a role in protecting DNA from single-strand breaks caused by free radicals in the body as well as a protective role in neurodegenerative diseases. As the end-product of purine degradation uric acid is generated in the xanthine/hypoxanthine reactions catalyzed by xanthine oxidase in humans, birds, new world monkeys, and some reptiles. Increased plasma concentrations of uric acid in selected species are also linked to the evolutionary loss of urate oxidase (the enzyme that oxidizes uric acid resulting in the formation of allantoin). It is the loss of uricase in association with increased uric acid concentrations that can be linked to a prolonged life span. The transcription and core promoter activity of XOR is repressed in humans, suggesting that there is a regulatory mechanism preventing the overproduction of uric acid associated with purine metabolism. Determination of such a relationship exists in species that lack the same Uox activity and whether this is, in fact, a coevolutionary event that can be linked to antioxidant defense involving uric acid is needed. In order to handle the metabolism of uric acid, birds package uric acid in protein vesicles in the proximal nephron with the insoluble uric acid crystals excreted along with fecal material from the cloaca. Increasing uric acid concentrations by feeding inosine can reduce oxidative stress whereas administration of allopurinol, which lowered uric acid concentrations, markedly increases oxidative stress. Collectively, these observations suggest that uric acid is the most significant factor in the amelioration of the oxidative burden in birds though the mechanism by which this antioxidant is regulated remains under investigation.

Chapter II – Uric acid (UA) was long regarded as waste product. Since the early 1990s, the nonenzymatic antioxidant properties of UA have received increasing attention. It is now recognized that it accounts for over half of the antioxidant activity in human blood. Most of the neuroprotective activity of UA is related to its ability to scavenge peroxynitrite-derived free radicals before they can react with their targeted biological molecules. Numerous observations and experimental data provide persuasive evidence for an altered metabolism of UA in diverse pathological states of the central nervous system (CNS) such as multiple sclerosis, optic neuritis, amyotrophic lateral sclerosis, Parkinson, Alzheimer, Huntington, Biswanger and variant Creutzfeld-Jakob diseases. This wide involvement of UA is likely due to the fact that oxidative stress and excitotoxicity are the final interacting pathways leading to cell death, and that UA is a major antioxidant which also reduces glutamate toxicity. The disturbances in UA metabolism are reflected by serum and cerebrospinal fluid (CSF) level changes. Most observations report lower UA serum values in multiple sclerosis and neurodegenerative diseases. CSF and brain tissue UA levels are found lower in most neurodegenerative diseases compared with healthy people. By contrast, in multiple sclerosis and Biswanger disease, where the blood brain barrier is altered, UA concentrations seem higher than in normal brain. Lower serum concentrations of UA may represent a primary, constitutive loss of protection against oxidative stress or a deficit secondary to UA consumption during oxidative radical scavenging. Higher concentrations of UA in CSF and brain may result from blood brain barrier leakage. Alternatively, they may reflect a rise in purine compounds degradation and consequently in their end product UA, due to an imbalance in ATP metabolism and energy state deficiency. In this hypothesis, UA would simply be an indirect marker of energy state imbalance. Despite convincing experimental and clinical data indicating a potential neuroprotective role for UA in multiple sclerosis, a thoroughly conducted, placebo-controlled, double blind clinical trial maintaining an asymptomatic hyperuricaemia for 2 years did not provide any benefit on accumulation of disability in relapsing-progressing MS patients. The negative results of this trial supplementing a single antioxidative molecule, compared with the positive results of a recent clinical study activating the Nrf2-ARE pathway, suggest that activation of a global neuroprotective pathway is more effective than supplementation of one of its components alone.

Chapter III –. Metabolic syndrome (MS) comprises pathological conditions that include insulin resistance, arterial hypertension, obesity and dyslipidemia; associated abnormalities include inflammation and endothelial dysfunction. Uric acid increase is considered an important risk factor for the development of cardiovascular disease favoring oxidative stress and endothelial dysfunction, thus being involved in MS pathophisiology. There is supporting evidence that uric acid may have a pathogenic role in the metabolic syndrome. Insulin has a physiologic action on renal tubules, causing a reduction in uric acid clearance, what could explain the higher uric acid levels found in MS. It was hypothesized a causal role of uric acid in fructose-induced metabolic syndrome showing that uric acid dose dependently blocked acethylcholine mediated arterial dilatation, suggesting that uric acid can impair endothelial function. In addition, it was verified that allopurinol, a xanthine oxidase inhibitor that lowers serum uric acid, was able to decrease systolic blood pressure, improve insulin sensitivity, and normalize triacylglycerol levels in fructose-induced metabolic syndrome. Moreover, uric acid can contribute to oxidative stress present in MS. Uric acid may trigger the reactive oxygen substances (ROS) generation through various mechanisms, for instance, activating the NADPH oxidase system. This statement was demonstrated in adypocites. ROS increase give raise to peroxinitrite ($ONOO^-$) by reaction with nitric oxide (NO) leading to protein nitrosylation, lipid peroxidation and NO• reduction altering endothelial function. Furthermore, uric acid has been shown to reduce NO bioavailability in various cell types via mechanisms involving redox control and also activating arginase and depleting NO. Uric acid can also form free radicals in various reactions, including peroxynitrite whose products are responsible for the amplification of lipid oxidation. However, it has also an important role in the antioxidant defense system. Uric acid is an important antioxidant, being responsible for 60% of the scavenging activity of the free radicals in human plasma. Uric acid reduces organic peroxyl radicals (ROO•) into hydroperoxide (ROOH), blockading its degradation to low molecular weight aldehydes. There is a positive correlation between uric acid levels and total antioxidant capacity. Therefore, uric acid seems to have a double role in oxidative stress measurements. Uric acid involvement in oxidative and nitroactive stress is very complex because its antioxidant/prooxidant capacity and probably this balance are concentration and pH dependent. Although uric acid may have a protective effect due to its antioxidant properties, it is clear that the dominant effect of uric acid in MS is deleterious. Long-term studies to verify the consequences of decreasing uric acid concentration below current recommendations in asymptomatic patients are needed.

Chapter IV – Clinical evidence suggests that hyperuricemia is an important, independent risk factor for cardiovascular renal disease and hypertension. A post-hoc analysis of hypertension clinical trials has also shown that patients with lower serum uric acid levels have a better outcome after reducing their blood pressure with anti-hypertensive drugs. Evidence from a cross-sectional study found that serum uric acid levels were significantly linear, corresponding to serum creatinine levels and suggesting that serum uric acid may play an intermediate role in reflecting renal function; this may be regarded as representing serum creatinine in renal failure progression in hypertensive subjects. Nevertheless, a recent animal study had demonstrated that uric acid may produce hypertension and renal failure by inducing vascular endothelial damage and produce vascular dysfunction, thus activating the renin angiotensin system. However, controversy exists, due to the lack of clinical evidence, to explore the causal effect between uric acid and hypertension development. Therefore, it is still not yet known whether serum uric acid is the cause or the marker of the hypertension and renal failure. Clinical trials are needed to determine if a uric acid lowering therapy would be effective in preventing renal failure and hypertension.

Chapter V – Uric acid is the end-product of the purine metabolism in human beings. Most of this substance is in the form of monosodium urate in compartments with pH 7.4 , such as plasma and extracellular fluids. In urine, where pH can be between 4.7 and 8.0, the ratio of uric acid - urate varies with pH, being this substance entirely as uric acid at acid urine: pH of 5.0 or less. Normal plasma uric acid level is 2.2–7.5 mg/dl in adult males, and it is slightly lower in premenopausal females: 2.1- 6.6 mg/dl. Normally, two-thirds of uric acid is eliminated by the kidney and one-third by the gut. Only 4 % of this substance is bound to plasma proteins, thus most of it is freely filterable and it can be dialyzed from plasma. Around 10 % of the filtrated urate is finally excreted in the urine. In the kidney, uric acid is mainly handled in the proximal tubule where it suffers two processes: reabsorption and secretion. In chronic renal disease serum urate increases at the same rate as creatinine, as creatininemia increases further the uricemia does not, because of an increase in its fractional excretion which can reach 85 % or more in advanced renal failure. Furthermore, there is an increased gut secretion of this substance in this setting. Regarding serum uric acid alterations: Hypouricemia is observed in the setting of uricosuric agents (benzbromarone), proximal tubular dysfunction, and syndrome of inappropriate antidiuretic hormone secretion, hematological malignant disorders and secondary to some drugs such as: corticosteroids, losartan, and low dose of non steroidal anti- inflammatories. Hyperuricemia is observed in gout inflammatory arthritis, acid uric urolithyasis, chronic renal disease, acute hyperuricemic nephropathy (tumoral lysis), and rhabdomyolysis. In conclusion, uric acid comes from purine metabolism, it is mainly excreted by the kidney and its serum levels can be altered by different conditions such as metabolic factors, drug influence, renal disease, and/or tissue destruction.

Chapter VI – This chapter deals with the positive association between serum UA and cardiovascular disease, which has been found not only in the high risk factor population but also in the general population. We summarize the association of UA within the literature and the underlying mechanisms of UA with cardiovascular disease in diabetic patients, starting with the antioxidant prooxidant UA redox shuttle, followed by the association between UA and inflammation. We also discuss prognostic implications of uric acid, urea and creatinin in diabetic patients, with cautionary notes about their clinical management

In: Uric Acid
Editors: S. Castillo and E. Maldonado
ISBN 978-1-62100-762-3

Chapter I

The Role of Uric Acid in the Avian Species

M. D. Carro[2], T. Settle[1], and H. Klandorf[1]
[1]Division of Animal and Nutrtional Sciences
West Virginia University, Morgantown,US
[2]Departamento de Producción Animal
Universidad de León, León, Spain

Abstract

Birds have a remarkable longevity for their body size despite an increased body temperature, higher metabolic rate, and increased blood glucose concentrations. Theoretically, birds should sustain a much higher degree of oxidative damage and processes leading to senescence such as glycoxidation of proteins and nucleic acids. Because this is not the case this suggests that birds have developed a more efficacious antioxidant defense system in order to cope with the oxidative burden. In actual fact birds have evolved into uric acid 'machines': uric acid is a potent antioxidant that is known to scavenge singlet oxygen, peroxy radicals, and hydroxyl radicals. Uric acid also binds with other primary radicals in addition to neutralizing iron ion complexes, which could signify additional antioxidant capabilities. Uric acid has a role in protecting DNA from single-strand breaks caused by free radicals in the body as well as a protective role in neurodegenerative diseases. As the end-product of purine degradation uric acid is generated in the xanthine/hypoxanthine reactions catalyzed by xanthine oxidase in humans, birds, new world monkeys, and some reptiles. Increased plasma concentrations of uric acid in selected species are also linked to the evolutionary loss of urate oxidase (the enzyme that oxidizes uric acid resulting in the formation of allantoin). It is the loss of uricase in association with increased uric acid concentrations that can be linked to a prolonged life span. The transcription and core promoter activity of XOR is repressed in humans, suggesting that there is a regulatory mechanism preventing the overproduction of uric acid associated with purine metabolism. Determination of such a relationship exists in species that lack the same Uox activity and whether this is, in fact, a coevolutionary event that can be linked to antioxidant defense involving uric acid is needed. In order to handle the metabolism of uric acid, birds package uric acid in protein vesicles in the proximal nephron with the insoluble uric acid crystals excreted along with fecal material from the cloaca. Increasing uric acid concentrations by feeding inosine can reduce oxidative stress whereas administration of allopurinol, which lowered uric acid concentrations, markedly increases oxidative stress. Collectively, these observations suggest that uric acid is the most significant factor in the amelioration of the oxidative burden in birds though the mechanism by which this antioxidant is regulated remains under investigation.

Introduction

Birds have a remarkable longevity for their body size despite an increased body temperature, higher metabolic rate, and increased blood glucose concentrations compared with mammals (Holmes and Austad, 1995). Theoretically, birds should sustain a much higher degree of oxidative damage and processes leading to senescence such as glycoxidation of proteins and nucleic acids (Monnier et al., 1991). For example a mouse that weighs approximately 20 g is equal in body size to a canary and yet the mouse will live 3 years as with one-twentieth the oxidative burden as opposed to the canary that will live 20 years (Holmes and Austad, 1995). This suggests that birds have developed effective mechanisms to cope with reactive oxygen species (ROS) assault by either reducing the amount of ROS produced or by a more efficient endogenous antioxidant defense system.

The production of endogenous ROS is associated with "leak" of electrons and protons from the electron transport chain in the mitochondria. Unlike short-lived vertebrates, most birds evidence a low mitochondrial ROS production. This has been measured in heart (Barja, 1998) and skeletal muscles responsible for flight (Suarez et al., 1991) in various species. A reduction in endogenous ROS production has also been linked to a decrease in oxidative stress and damage in birds. This link has implications in the aging process of birds. Most birds have a substantial longevity despite heightened metabolic demands as compared to mammals of comparable body size (Munshi-South and Wilkinson, 2009). However, despite a low mitochondrial ROS production there is cumulative oxidative damage by ROS throughout the lifespan of the bird. To cope with this production of ROS over time, birds must capitalize on a more efficient antioxidant defense system.

Like other species, birds rely on exogenous and endogenous antioxidant defense systems. The exogenous antioxidants are obtained primarily from the diet and other environmental factors. Endogenous antioxidants include superoxide dismutase, glutathione peroxidase, estrogen, and uric acid. Uric acid is a potent antioxidant and it is, arguably, the dominant antioxidant defense mechanism for birds (Seaman et al., 2008, Stinefelt et al., 2005, Machin et al., 2004, Simoyi et al., 2002, Klandorf et al., 2001). Uric acid is the end product of purine degradation in birds. Due to the evolutionary lack of urate oxidase expression, also known as uricase, birds (comparable to reptiles, higher primates, and humans) do not convert uric acid to allantoin.

The enzyme xanthine oxidoreductase (XOR) catalyzes the reaction between hypoxanthine and xanthine to form uric acid. This enzyme is present in two forms: xanthine dehydrogenase (XD) and xanthine oxidase (XO). In birds, XD is the predominant form in the liver, kidney, pancreas, intestine, and other tissues (Harrison, 2002). Recently, however, XO activity has been measured in chicken liver, kidney, pancreas, and intestine (Carro et al., 2009a).

The purpose of this review is to examine the role of uric acid as an antioxidant defense mechanism in birds against free radical damage and how this ultimately contributes to longevity in birds.

Avian Mitochondria: Structure and ROS Production

The mitochondrion has been described as the "powerhouse" of the cell. This is due to the electron transport chain that results in the release of energy and the proton pumps that result in energy conservation through oxidative phosphorylation. The mitochondria are composed of an outer membrane, the inner membrane, cristae, and matrix. The inner membrane is folded into cristae, which markedly increases the surface area. It is within the inner membrane that the enzyme complexes for electron transport and oxidative phosphorylation reside as well as other transfer systems and various dehydrogenase enzymes. The matrix contains enzymes for fatty acid oxide-tion, urea synthesis, prophoryin synthesis, and the tricarboxylic acid cycle (TCA) in addition to other processes. The mitochondrial DNA (mtDNA), ribosomes, and proteins necessary for transcription of mtDNA and translation of mRNA are also found within the matrix. These basic structures are found throughout the animal kingdom for those animals that rely on oxygen as the final electron acceptor.

Birds, while sharing the same basic mitochondrial structure with mammalian and reptilian species, also exhibit some unique differences. Slautterback (1965) was the first to note a difference in avian mitochondrial structure. In this study, mitochondria were isolated from the cardiac cells of canaries, sparrows, zebra finches, quail, and geese. Species were selected on the basis of heart rate. For example, canaries, sparrows, and zebra finches have a very fast heart rate whereas the quail and goose have an intermediate and slower heart rate, respectively. Surprisingly, mitochondria from the canary cardiac tissue showed two unique structures of cristae, referred to as zigzag and the others as retriform. These names were assigned to each structure based on the appearance of the cristae patterns. Quail cardiac mitochondria also demonstrated numerous and tightly packed interleaved cristae with a much greater length than the width. Also present in the quail were whorl patterns of cristae. The goose model, with the lower heart rate, revealed fewer and less complex cristae. From these results it was concluded that there was a poor correlation between heart rate and the complexity or size of cardiac mithochondria in birds. However, the findings of unique mitochondrial morphologies between the species created a foundation for further research into various tissues with an emphasis on skeletal muscles used for flight.

Research into flight muscles of hummingbirds revealed that the mitochondrial structure differs from that of other vertebrates. Hummingbirds are unique in that the respiration rates of flight muscle range from 7-10 mL of O_2 per cm^3 of mitochondria per minute, nearly twice that of mammals moving at maximum aerobic capacity (Suarez et al., 1991). This phenomenon is achieved by a double packing of mitochondrial cristae (Suarez et al., 1991). It is also remarkable that mitochondria occupy about 35% of the fiber volume in hummingbird flight muscles; mammals, in contrast, would require approximately 70% mitochondrial volume to achieve this respiratory rate, which would not be sufficient to provide lift due to lack of force-generating myofibrils (Rome and Lindstedt, 1998). These structural differences in avian mitochondria give rise to a greater ability to more efficiently utilize oxygen.

Mitochondrial Generation of ROS

Mitochondria are responsible for the leakage of high energy electron via the electron transport chain in a normal metabolic state (Fig.1). Complex III is the principal site for production of ROS as the ROS products are directed away from the matrix antioxidants whereas ROS products in complex I are released in proximity to antioxidants (Chen et al., 2003). Complex II and complex IV are also implicated in ROS production, specifically concerning the superoxide anion and has been reviewed extensively by Turrens (2003).

Reactive oxygen species are free radicals derived from molecular oxygen with an unpaired electron. Oxygen is required for the generation of all ROS and reactive nitrogen species (RNS) as well as reactive chlorine species (Fang et al., 2002). Ground state oxygen, also referred to as the triplet state, is considered to be a bi-radical, meaning that it contains two unpaired electrons in the outer shell. The two electrons exhibit the same spin which enables the oxygen molecule to react with one electron at a time. In a chemical bond, oxygen is not particularly reactive with the two electrons. However, if one of the unpaired electrons becomes excited it can alter its spin pattern which results in a singlet oxygen species. The singlet oxygen can react with other pairs of electrons, especially those involved in double bonds, which can transform into a powerful oxidant (Halliwell and Gutteridge, 1999). ROS can hold a dual nature, either beneficial to the immune response or detrimental in cases of overproduction of ROS.

The most commonly known ROS produced in biological systems include the hydroxyl radical (·OH), the superoxide radical ($O_2^{-}\cdot$), nitric oxide (NO·), peroxynitrite ($ONOO^{-}$), and hydrogen peroxide (H_2O_2). Free radicals and other ROS are constantly formed in the body and have been implicated in patogenic states and oxidative stress (Aruoma, 1998). Of these ROS, superoxide and hydrogen peroxide radicals are of the most importance in reduction-oxidation reactions as well as substrates in the formation of other ROS, particularly the highly toxic hydroxyl radical (Halliwell and Gutteridge, 1999).

Hydroxyl radicals (·OH) can attack all proteins, DNA, polyunsaturated fatty acids (PUFA) in cell membranes, and a variety of other molecules (Aruoma, 1998). Hydroxyl radicals can be generated by Fenton chemistry ($Fe^{2+} + H_2O \rightarrow Fe^{3+} + {}^{\cdot}OH + {}^{-}OH$), which are catalyzed by transition metals.

Fenton reaction generation of OH· radicals is known to occur in submitochondrial particles under oxidative stress (Thomas et al., 2009) as well as during a number of toxicological states (Hara et al., 2009). Exposure to radiation can cause homolytic fission of water molecules, resulting in the generation of hydroxyl radicals as well (Halliwell and Gutteridge, 1999). Reduction-oxidation reactions with superoxide, hydrogen peroxide, and hypochlorous acid also generate hydroxyl radicals *in vivo* (Rosen et al., 1995).

Superoxide radicals are normally produced in the body via respiratory burst during phagocytosis in immunological defense and from the leakage of electrons from the mitochondrial electron transport chain. Superoxide is an oxygen-centered radical and can have selective reactivity to a variety of tissue types, proteins, DNA, etc. (Aruoma, 1998). In addition to superoxide radicals, hydrogen peroxide is produced during mitochondrial respiration and during xanthine/hypoxanthine reaction associated with purine degradation (Terada et al., 1990). H_2O_2 can also be formed when superoxide is dismutated (a reaction involving a single substance that produces two products) by the enzyme superoxide dismutase, although in comparison to superoxide is less reactive (Aruoma, 1998). However, H_2O_2 can act as a substrate for hydroxyl radical production as well as generation of other ROS.

Avian Mitochondrial ROS Production

Given that birds have double-packed cristae, it is of interest to determine how this affects ROS production. Surprisingly, birds have a lower mitochondrial ROS production rate. Hydrogen peroxide production was lower in brain tissue mitochondria of pigeons than in rats (Barja et al., 1994). Additional studies in the nonsynaptic neural mitochondria of pigeons indicated that ROS production was less in complex I as compared to ROS production in the same tissue of rats (Barja and Herrero, 1998). Further studies with brain mitochondrial complex I in budgerigar and canaries showed similar results, with comparatively lowered ROS production (Pamplona et al., 2005). Mitochondrial hydrogen peroxide release rate was also lower in the brain, heart, and kidney of pigeons as compared to rats (Barja, 1998).

Recently, Brown et al. (2009) proposed a mechanism responsible for the reduction of ROS production in birds. Mitochondria from the livers of House sparrows (*Passer domesticus*), the big brown bat (*Eptesicus fuscus*), and mice (*Mus musculus*) were isolated for analysis of mitochondrial respiration rates, proton leak kinetics, and hydrogen peroxide release. Basal hydrogen peroxide rates were two-fold higher in the sparrows compared to the mice, while inhibition of the electron transport chain with rotenone and antimycin A increased ROS production rate by 20-27 fold in sparrows as compared to mice (Brown et al., 2009). These results are consistent with the hypothesis of "spare oxidative capacity" put forth by Lane (2005), which predicts higher substrate oxidation capacity downstream of ROS production sites (relative to upstream capacity). Consequently, electron transport chain reduction state is reduced, as is ROS release rate in birds. It can thus be concluded that there are distinct mechanisms by which ROS release from the mitochondria is controlled and that these mechanisms are species specific.

Oxidative Stress

The ground state of oxygen is essential to all aerobic organisms. However, oxygen reliance can lead to toxicity and imbalance in the body's physiological processes.

Oxidative stress is defined as the imbalance between the oxidants (ROS) in the body and the antioxidants such that the imbalance favors the oxidants (VanDyke et al., 2002). The ROS imbalance can be caused, in general, by diminished antioxidant protection or by increased production of ROS (Halliwell and Gutteridge, 1999). This can be caused by endogenous sources such as the leak of electrons from the mitochondria (Cadenas and Davies, 2000) and exogenous sources such as pollutants (Hara et al., 2009), radiation, and other environmental factors. Accumulated damage by ROS contributes to many pathogenic states, as well as non-pathogenic states, and is due to the highly unstable nature of the ROS. Strand breakage, base modification, and DNA-protein crosslinks can be linked to ROS mediated damage (Halliwell and Gutteridge, 1999). Accumulation of damage by ROS results in a condition known as oxidative stress.

Oxidative stress has been implied as one of the major contributing factors damage resulting in to DNA. In response, DNA repair mechanisms function *in vivo* continuously (Aruoma, 1998). Hydroxyl and superoxide radicals are implicated in the mechanism behind DNA damage. However, single strand-breaks of DNA can be inhibited by antioxidant defense systems such as uric acid (Cohen et al., 1984).

Oxidative stress has also been associated with various disease states such as ischemia and reperfusion injury, diabetes, and neurodegenerative disorders.

Ischemia reperfusion injury occurs during cardiovascular events or damage to the brain in which the tissue is deprived of oxygen (Halliwell and Gutteridge, 1999). Associated with these events is an increase in both ROS and XOR activity, which leads to a release of superoxide radicals as a consequence of the reaction with xanthine (Harrison, 2002). It has also been reported that peroxynitrite has a role in central nervous system (CNS) inflammation (Hooper et al., 2000) and in multiple sclerosis (Hooper et al., 1998).

Oxidative stress is also a factor in the aging process (Fig. 1). Over time, oxidative damage has an effect on glycoxidation of proteins, lipids, and DNA. These markers can accumulate over time and have an impact on aging (Beckman and Ames, 1998). A study by Pamplona et al. (2005) demonstrated that protein and lipid oxidative damage were lower in brain mitochondria of budgerigars and canaries when compared to mice. Birds are considered a long-lived species. Given what is known about the lowered endogenous ROS production in birds along with the suggestion that there are lowered states of oxidative damage, the link between these factors and aging needs to be determined. Based on the Free Radical Theory of Aging, senescence is a result of the accumulation of free radical induced oxidative damage over time (Beckman and Ames, 1998). In response, birds have developed a strategy to cope with free radical production that includes a reduction in mitochondrial ROS production (despite having double-packed cristae) along with a highly efficient antioxidant defense system. Con-sequently, birds have a reduced production of ROS from the mitochondrial electron transport chain associated with a decrease in oxidative damage. However, there remains the issue of heightened metabolism, elevated plasma glucose, and increased body temperature that are associated with oxidative damage sustained over time. It is thus essential that a long-lived species evolve an efficient antioxidant defense system. Birds, like humans, have a high concentration of uric acid circulating in the blood plasma. It has been hypothesized that, with the evolutionary loss of uricase, the enzyme responsible for the conversion of uric acid to allantoin, birds have become equipped with a very potent antioxidant defense.

The Evolutionary Loss of Uricase: Implications for Avian Longevity

Uric acid is the end-product of purine metabolism in humans, reptiles, new world primates, and birds. Unlike most mammals, these species lack uricase or urate oxidase (Uox) which catalyzes the oxidation of uric acid to allantoin. Analysis of the promoter coding exonic and intronic regions of human and several primate species determined that the hominoid lineage has eight independent nonsense mutations that resulted in the deactivation of the Uox gene (Oda et al., 2002). Of the eight mutations, six are caused by a change from C to T in the arginine codon (CGA). After examination of the prevalence of the arginine codon in the primate species, it was suggested that the increasing occurrence of the CGA codon is highly correlated with the loss of urate oxidase (Oda et al., 2002). The authors concluded that this loss was a stepwise event and not a single step over evolutionary time (Oda et al., 2002). Currently, the DNA database does not have a Uox sequence for birds or reptiles and further analysis will be needed to discover the reason for the evolutionary loss of Uox in these species. The fortuitous loss of this enzyme by long-lived species is considered to be linked to the antioxidant properties of uric acid. It is also hypothesized that coevolution occurred between the down regulation of XOR and the increase in uric acid concentrations in species lacking urate oxidase (Oda et al., 2002). The transcription and core promoter activity of human XOR is repressed (Xu et al., 2000), suggesting that there is a regulatory mechanism preventing the overproduction of uric acid associated with purine metabolism. It should be determined if such a relationship exists in species other than humans that lack the same Uox activity and whether this is, in fact, a coevolutionary event that can be linked to antioxidant defense involving uric acid. A review of the loss of uricase and clinical implications in human pathology has been written by Alvarez-Lario and Macarron-Vicente (2010)

Xanthine Oxidoreductase: The Formation of Uric Acid

XOR Chemistry and Structure

The enzyme XOR catalyzes the terminal reactions in purine degradation to uric acid. Specifically, XOR catalyzes the formation of uric acid from hypoxanthine and xanthine. This enzyme has been known for over 100 years and studied in detail for approximately 60 years (Harrison, 2002). XOR is a complex and highly conserved molybdoflavoenzyme, most notably found in bovine milk where it forms a major component of the milk fat globule membrane (Harrison, 2002). XOR exists in two interconvertible forms: XD (xanthine dehydrogenase) and XO (xanthine oxidase). XO catalyzes reactions (1) and (2), while XD catalyzes reaction (3) (Terada et al., 1990).

xanthine + $2O_2$ + H2O ↔ uric acid + $2O_2^-$ + 2 H +
(1)

xanthine + O_2 +H_2 O ↔ uric acid + H_2O_2
(2)

xanthine + NAD^+ +H_2O ↔ uric acid + NADH + H^+
(3)

The structure of XOR is considered to be a homodimer containing catalytically independent subunits with an approximate molecular mass of 300kDa and containing one molybdenum co–factor (Mo-Co), an FAD group, and two iron-sulfur centers. The protein structure of XO is comparatively large, having a molecular weight of 275,000 g/mol (Hart et al, 1970) while the protein structure of XD has a molecular weight of 300,000 g/mol (Lyon and Garret, 1978).

The oxidative hydroxylation of xanthine to uric acid occurs at the molybdenum center (Hille and Nishino, 1995). XO and XD differ in that XD can reduce both molecular oxygen and NAD^+ but has a greater affinity for the latter, while XO reacts only with molecular oxygen. Both forms catalyze the reaction which converts hypoxanthine to xanthine and then the further conversion of xanthine to uric acid. A complete understanding of the XOR reaction with xanthine remains uncertain in some aspects, although there are common features associated with this interaction. For example, the reaction of XOR with xanthine occurs as both a reduction and oxidation reaction (Xia et al., 1999).

The reductive half reaction occurs at the Mo-Co center. XOR accepts two electrons from xanthine, which reduces the Mo (VI) to Mo (IV). At the xanthine C8 position, hydrogen is transferred to a sulphido ligand of molybdenum which results in the conversion M=S bond into an M-SH bond. Simultaneously, there is a nucleophilic attack by a hydroxyl group at C8 which results in the formation of uric acid. The hydroxyl is ultimately derived from water, but it is uncertain if it reacts independently or as a Mo ligand (Murray et al., 1966).

The oxidative half reaction takes place at the FAD portion of the XOR molecule. The intramolecular electron transfer between the Mo-Co and FAD is mediated by the Fe_2-S_2 center (Hille and Anderson, 1991). The Fe_2-S_2 center serves as an electron reservoir to maintain the Mo-Co as Mo (VI) and flavin as $FADH_2$ for the reaction catalysis (Olson et al., 1974). Electrons are transferred from FAD to NAD^+ or O_2. In the reoxidation of fully reduced XO, the first two steps involve the transfer of two electrons to O_2, which generate hydrogen peroxide (Berry and Hare, 2004; Hille and Massey, 1981). XO transfers its remaining electrons in separate steps which results in the independent reduction of O_2 from which superoxides are formed (Berry and Hare, 2004). The overall oxidation reaction of XO yields two superoxide radicals and two peroxides.

In comparison to XO, XD may produce more superoxide radicals in reaction per mole of O_2. This occurs as a result of the greater thermodynamic stability of FAD, which is more reactive with oxygen in the XD form. While XD may produce more superoxide radicals, XD reacts more slowly with oxygen: the maximal rate of superoxide production is 25% less than that of XO (Saito and Nishino, 1989). This may also be due to the greater affinity of NAD^+ binding with XD, making O_2 a poor competitor (Harris and Massy, 1997). The mechanism of electron transfer from XD to NAD^+ is not as well understood as that of oxygen, but it is suggested that XD cycles between a two and a four electron-reduced state (Harris and Massey, 1997). NAD^+ binds to XD in the reduction of the four electron state and subsequently transfers two electrons to produce NADH (Harris and Massey, 1997). Detailed reviews of this mechanism have been published by Harris (2002) and Hille and Nishino (1995).

XOR has been implicated in various pathological states due to the increased production of ROS (superoxide, hydroxyl, and hydrogen peroxide). The production of these ROS results in increased oxidative stress within the organism, which increases the instance of disease particularly if the endogenous antioxidant protection is somehow compromised. In the case of XOR, the enzyme is thought to play a role in tissue structural damage and inter-ference of cell signaling (Berry and Hare, 2004).

The gene structure of XOR has been determined in several species including humans, mice, chickens, and insects. The gene loci that code for human and mouse XOR have been elucidated and the associated genes have been assigned to chromosomes 2p22 and 17 (Harrison, 2002; Cazzaniga et al., 1994). *Drosophila* genes tend to be more compact with only four or five exons (Terao et al., 1997). In mammals the exon-intron structure is highly conserved with approximately 36 exons (Xu et al., 1996). Mammalian and avian cDNA sequences have also been reported. Avians, specifically chickens, have a sequence that corresponds to 1358 amino acids whereas mammalian enzymes range from 1330-1335 amino acids with 90% homology (Harrison, 2002). The Mo-Co binding site is the most conserved of the amino acid sequences and has a 94% homology between human, rat, and mouse XOR (Xu et al., 1995).

Mutations in the XOR gene in humans, more specifically concerning the XD form, have been linked to inheritable xanthinuria. Classic xanthinuria is categorized into two different types: type I xanthinuria is characterized by the lack of XD activity whereas type II is characterized by the lack of both XD and aldehyde oxidase. Several mutations have been found to be responsible for the type I condition, including a point mutation from C to T in nucleotide 445 which changed the codon from Arg to Cys (Sakamoto et al., 2001). The mutations associated with type II have been located on the gene for human molybdenum cofactor sulphurase, which is required for XOR activity (Ichida et al., 2001). The majority of patients with xanthinuria present as asymptomatic, while others present with renal failure, xanthine calculi, and excretion of xanthine in the urine.

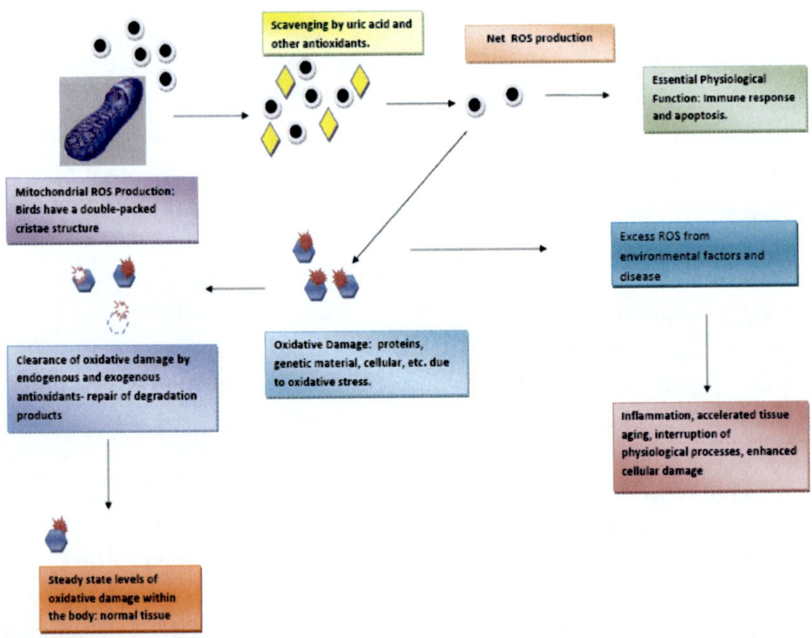

Figure 1. Schematic of mitochondrial reactive oxygen species (ROS) production, antioxidant defense, and oxidative stress. As adapted from Terzioglu and Larsson (2007).

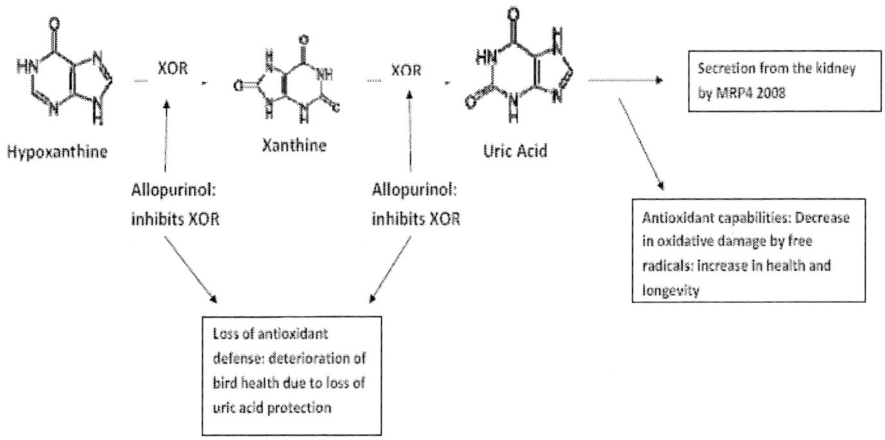

Figure 2. Normal and inhibited uric acid formation with implications to bird health and oxidative stress. Role of allopurinol in the inhibition of xanthine oxidoreductase (XOR).

XOR activity can be inhibited by allopurinol (1,5 dihydro-4-hydroxypyrazolo [3,4-d] pyrimidin-4-one) and oxypurinol (Figure 2). Allopurinol is the structural analog of hypoxanthine, meaning that it is chemically similar, however it has different biochemical properties. More specifically, it interferes with purine catabolism by inhibiting XOR. Allopurinol is rapidly oxidized by XOR *in vivo* to the active metabolite, oxypurinol (Pacher et al., 2006).

Both allopurinol and oxypurinol are isosteres (have the same number of valence electrons) of hypoxanthine and xanthine respectively (Pacher et al., 2006). Allopurinol binds to Mo (VI) and is oxidized while oxypurinol binds to Mo (IV) and is reduced. The reduced XOR-oxypurinol complex rearranges into a tightly bound inhibitory complex (Galbusera et al., 2006). Oxypurinol is a noncompetitive inhibitor of XOR while allopurinol can act as a competitive inhibitor at low concentrations and noncompetitive at high concentrations (Pacher et al., 2006). Allopurinol can be administered either orally or by intravenous injection (Pea, 2005). Evidence suggests that allopurinol has a half life of 2-3h and reaches peak plasma concentrations 30-60 min following oral dosage. Oral bioavailability of allopurinol is suggested to be 67-90% (Pea, 2005). Oxypurinol has a lower oral bioavailability than allopurinol with a half life of 14-30h which is thought to be due to a reduced renal absorption resulting in peak plasma concentration occurring in 3-5h (Pea, 2005).

Mammalian XOR Tissue Distribution

XOR activity has been detected in a number of mammalian species as well as bacteria and plants. XOR activity in mammalian species has been found to be highest in the liver and intestine (Harrison, 2002; Parks and Granger, 1986). There is also evidence of enzyme activity in the heart, pancreas, brain, kidney and blood plasma. In reptiles, XOR activity has been reported in the kidney tissue of Dhubb lizards (Al-Seeni, 2009). Histochemical studies have given rise to evidence that the enzyme is present in the endothelial cells of bovine capillary and mammary glands (Jarasch et al., 1981), primarily in the cytosol of these cells. These locations were confirmed in humans (Jarasch et al., 1984). XOR activity in both forms has also been located in epithelia of a variety of rat tissues. Moriwaki and colleagues (1998) measured XOR activity in rat tissues using an immunohistochemical technique developed by Kooij et al. (1991). The findings of this study demonstrated a comparatively increased enzyme activity in the small intestine and moderate activity in the surface epithelium of the tongue, esophagus, stomach, bronchioles, alveoli, renal tubules, and large intestine. Activity was also moderate to strong in the liver, particularly in the cytoplasm of the hepatic and sinusoidal cells and with greater activity in the pericentral zone of these cells (Moriwaki et al., 1998). A biochemical study by Devenyi et al. (1987) found XOR activity, in the XD form, in the pancreatic tissue of control mice as well as XO activity in the pancreatic homogenate, which was contributed to the reversible conversion of XD to XO.

Along with tissue distribution, the subcellular localization of XOR is not yet fully understood in mammalian models. Some studies have suggested that the XOR is found predominately in the cytosol of endothelial cells of bovine tissue and rat hepatocytes (Jarasch et al., 1984; Ischikawa et al., 1992). Other studies have suggested various locations for both forms of XOR, including the peroxisomes of rat hepatocytes (Angermuller et al., 1987), on the cell membrane surface and the cytosol of human endothelial and epithelial cells (Rouquette et al., 1998), and in the pericentral zone of the cytoplasm in hepatic rat cells (Moriwaki et al., 1998). Research to determine the tissue distribution and the localization of XOR within the cell environment is thus still needed.

Evidence for an antibody specific to XOR has been discovered in the blood of humans and other mammals. A study by Chen et al. (1996) found that XOR was virtually absent from the plasma of sheep and cattle, but was present in the plasma of buffalo. A study by Benboubetra and colleagues (1997) concluded that there were both IgG and IgM antibodies specific to XOR. A previous study by Bruder et al., (1984) concluded that IgG antibodies were present in rabbit, guinea pig, goat, bovine, mouse, and human sera; however, there is no known immune memory generated over multiple exposure to XOR or immunological tolerance to this protein (Bruder et al, 1984), suggesting that there is no immunity to circulating XOR.

Avian XOR Tissue Distribution

Similar to mammals, avian XOR is predominately found in the XD form with low, but detectable levels of XO activity. XOR has been studied extensively in the XD form in chickens and turkeys. XOR, in the XD form was first described as being non-autoxidizable in birds, which would differ from mammalian XO (Westerfeld and Richert, 1951). Subsequent studies have focused on a variety of variables that could affect XOR activity in birds including nutrition trials with variable protein content, starvation and re-feeding, and embryonic development.

Results from nutrition trials showed that as protein content increases in the diet, XOR activity also increases. Westerfeld et al. (1962) reported that soy and casein diets fed to chicks and poults increased XD activity in liver tissue in a relatively linear relationship with protein content with no significant difference between the sources of protein. Scholz and Featherston (1967) reported that an increase in isolated soybean protein in the diet (25 or 75%) increased XD activity in the liver of 21-day old chicks and also resulted in an increased enzyme activity after a 24 hour starvation period.

In addition to nutritional studies, XOR activity has also been measured in birds administered allopurinol (Fhaolain and Coughlan, 1978) or inosine (Della-Corte and Stirpe, 1967). Turkey liver samples incubated with allopurinol resulted in a progressive loss of XD activity until less than 1% remained after three minutes (Fhaolain and Coughlan, 1978). Recently, Carro et al. (2009b) found that XOR activity in the liver tissue of broilers administered allopurinol (50 mg/kg body mass) was significantly increased and concluded that this could be a compensatory mechanism to maintain normal uric acid concentrations in the body. Feeding a mixture of allopurinol and inosine (a purine precursor) to chickens for 6 days, caused a significant decrease in liver XOR activity and uric acid concentrations in the liver tissue, indicating that the allopurinol was inhibiting XOR activity regardless of the presence of inosine which is converted into uric acid (Settle et al, unpublished data; see Table 1).

Table 1. Effects of feeding inosine (161 g of inosine/kg feed) and inosine plus allopurinol (161 g of inosine plus 0.5 g of allopurinol/kg feed) on activities of xanthine oxidase (XO) and xanthine dehydrogenase (XD) and uric acid concentration in the liver of broilers (n=5)

	Activity (units/mg protein)				Uric acid	
Treatment	XO	XD	XO + XD	Total XO + XD activity (units/liver)	mg/g wet tissue	total mg in the liver
Control	7.92	37.9	45.9	24.7 [b]	0.262 [b]	15.5 [b]
Inosine	7.97	37.2	44.6	20.9 [ab]	0.266 [b]	14.3 [b]
Inosine + allopurinol	7.33	35.7	43.7	16.2 [a]	0.093 [a]	3.76 [a]
SEM	0.559	2.50	3.00	1.49	0.0333	1.582
P =	0.673	0.812	0.875	0.005	0.005	< 0.001

[a, b] For each variable, means within a column lacking a common superscript differ ($P<0.05$).

SEM: standard error of the mean.

XOR activity has also been measured during the development of the embryo and immediately after hatching. It was noted that XD increases significantly in the liver for at least eight days prior to hatching and after hatch (Strittmatter, 1965). Additionally, chick embryos showed detectable amounts of XD at approximately 10 days of development (Strittmatter, 1965). Embryonic leg and breast muscle tissue showed detectable XOR activity at 10 days of development, which peaked in breast muscle at hatch (Garcia-Palmer et al., 1985).

Remy et al. (1951) and Nishino et al. (1989) also reported that XOR was present in chicken liver and kidney tissue although XO was a minor component of the total XOR activity. However, the majority of the earlier studies did not specifically measure XO activity. Carro et al. (2009a) reported that detectable XO activity was found in the liver, pancreas, kidney, intestine, and breast muscle in 7 and 10-week old broilers while no activity was found either in the plasma or in the heart, brain, or lung tissues. XD was the predominant form of XOR in all tissues, but XD activity was much lower in the breast muscle, brain, heart, and lungs than in the rest of the analyzed tissues.

Uric Acid in the Antioxidant Defense System

Organisms balance their redox status by antioxidant inactivation of ROS. An antioxidant is, broadly, an agent that catalytically scavenges ROS and reactive RNS (Halliwell and Gutteridge, 1999). Antioxidants tend to work at low concentrations and are readily oxidized by ROS thereby limiting the ability of ROS to react with the surrounding cells and tissues.

Uric acid is known to scavenge singlet oxygen, peroxy radicals, and hydroxyl radicals (Ames et al., 1981). Uric acid interacts with iron ion complexes, in that it exhibits an ability to bind these complexes which could signify additional antioxidant capabilities (Davies et al., 1986). Uric acid also has a role in protecting DNA from single-strand breaks caused by free radicals in the body (Cohen et al., 1984) as well as a protective role in neurodegenerative diseases. Uric acid, as a scavenger of peroxynitrite, has been shown to exhibit protective properties in the inhibition of CNS inflammation and the blood-CNS barrier that has been compromised by peroxynitrite damage (Hooper et al., 2000). In addition to this, uric acid treatment in a mouse model for encephalomyelitis resulted in a significant reduction in the symptoms and increased survivability (Hooper et al., 1998). In contrast, increased uric acid concentrations are linked with cardiovascular disease and are a well known painful complication of gout when excretion is impaired (Skinner et al., 1998).

Uric acid is the dominant antioxidant defense system for birds and can be linked to their ability to cope with the heightened metabolic ROS production throughout their lives. The concentration of uric acid in broiler plasma ranges from 0.2 to 0.8 mM (Simoyi et al., 2002). A study by Stinefelt et al. (2005), using electron spin resonance, demonstrated the free radical scavenging abilities of uric acid, in doses equal to and exceeding the physiological range found in birds. It was found that uric acid had a concentration-dependent effect on reducing generation such that increasing the concentration of uric acid resulted in an increased scavenging of these radicals (Stinefelt et al., 2005). This study also showed a decrease in DNA fragmentation and lipid peroxidation (Stinefelt et al., 2005), which supports the view that uric acid acts as a potent scavenger of free radicals and is essential to antioxidant defense in birds.

In addition, there are several studies with chickens that demonstrate a direct correlation between increased uric acid concentrations and a reduction in oxidative stress and vice versa. Broilers fed a high protein diet consisting of 45% casein had a significant increase in plasma uric acid concentrations, which was also associated with a decrease in oxidative stress in the fast growing birds suggesting that the protein levels were not detrimental to bird health (Machin et al., 2004). When broilers were fed diets containing either xanthine or hypoxanthine, plasma uric acid was increased as compared to controls and was associated with a decrease in oxidative stress (Simoyi et al., 2002). Alternatively, birds fed allopurinol (40 - 50 mg/kg body mass) showed decreased plasma uric acid concentrations associated with a significant increase in oxidative stress at both doses (Simoyi et al., 2002). A similar study with inosine (0.6M /kg feed/day) administered to broilers treated with hemin (a prooxidant) showed that inosine elevated plasma uric acid concentrations and reduced hemin-induced oxidative stress (Seaman et al., 2008). When a mixture of inosine and allopurinol were fed to broilers, there was a marked decrease in plasma and tissue uric acid concentrations as compared with broilers receiving only inosine, which suggests that tissues in treated animals may be more susceptible to oxidative damage (Settle et al, unpublished observations; see Table 2).

Table 2. Effects of feeding inosine (161 g of inosine/kg feed) and inosine plus allopurinol (161 g of inosine plus 0.5 g of allopurinol/kg feed) on plasma uric acid concentrations in broilers (n=5)

	Plasma uric acid (mg/dL)		
Treatment	Day 0	Day 3	Day 6
Control	5.12	4.41 [a]	4.46 [a]
Inosine	4.93	18.6 [c]	14.3 [b]
Inosine + allopurinol	4.96	13.9 [b]	12.0 [b]
SEM	0.530	1.070	1.133
P =	0.847	< 0.001	< 0.001

[a, b, c] For each variable, means within a column lacking a common superscript differ ($P<0.05$).
SEM: standard error of the mean.

Uric acid has also been studied in wild bird populations. Recently, Cohen et al. (2007) measured total antioxidant capacity, uric acid concentrations, and oxidative stress in 92 species of birds. The results from this study indicated that as the duration of captivity increase, so did oxidative stress, concomitant with a reduction in uric acid concentrations in the blood (Cohen et al., 2007). It was concluded that antioxidant activity decreased over time in response to the stress and was either being consumed or shunted from the bloodstream (Cohen et al., 2007). Conclusions from this study support the view that the inverse relationship between uric acid concentrations and oxidative stress are consistent across species. Uric acid is suggested to be the most important factor in the amelioration of oxidative burden in birds. Results from numerous studies have shown a correlation between the increase in plasma uric acid concentrations and a reduction in oxidative stress. In view of this observation, further research is critical for understanding the regulation of uric acid production in health and disease with the view to reduce oxidative burden.

Avian Renal Transport of Uric Acid

In birds uric acid is packaged in protein vesicles in the kidney before secretion (Braun and Dantzler, 1997) and the insoluble uric acid crystals are excreted along with fecal material from the cloaca (Skinner et al., 2001). Uric acid is secreted from the avian renal proximal tubule epithelium. A micropuncture study with European starlings (*Sturnus vulgaris*) determined the net flow and transport of urate by the nephron (Laverty and Dantzler, 1983). A fractional secretion rate of 4.72 on average was determined for starlings. Net urate secretion has also been measured in the chicken (Shannon, 1983) and ducks (Stewart et al., 1969) with a measured fractional secretion range of 6-16 percent. These studies suggest that urate transport is species specific and that birds have comparatively increased active transport of uric acid across the nephron and glomerulous. A more recent study by Dudas et al. (2005) in chicken renal proximal epithelium cell culture showed a secretion of [C^{14}] urate under control conditions in an Ussing Chamber to be at a ratio of 3:1. OAT 1, OAT3, MRP4, and MRP2, known transporters of human urate, were identified in the basolateral membrane and the brush border membrane of the renal tissue (Dudas et al., 2005). Further study of MRP4 in chick kidney tissues revealed that the transporter was present in the brush border membrane and that it is required for active urate secretion from the proximal tube epithelium (Bataille et al., 2008).

Avian Gout

While uric acid is a major antioxidant defense for birds, it can also be implicated in disease. Birds can suffer from hyperuricemia, a state during which uric acid precipitates in tissues of affected animals. Gout can be caused by several factors such as renal disorders, over supplementation of protein in the diet, and other causes (Lumeij et al., 1998). Avian gout exists in two forms: articular and visceral. Articular gout occurs when the crystals settle within the joints and, like gout in humans, is considered to be a chronic condition over time. This can lead to damage of the joint and thereby difficulty in movement and ultimately can lead to death due to inability to obtain food. Visceral gout is the more acute form in which the crystallized uric acid precipitates into the viscera causing extensive tissue damage that leads to organ failure and eventual death.

Susceptibility to articular gout was first identified in a specific strain of New Hampshire chickens with inherited muscular dystrophy when fed a high protein diet (80%) for a maximum 1-2 weeks of age, respectively (Peterson et al., 1971). There were no signs of gout in control birds. Visceral gout was not detected in any of the birds. Of note, XD activity in the liver was significantly increased in gout-susceptible birds, which was to be expected as it is one of two forms of the XOR enzyme responsible for uric acid production (Peterson et al., 1971). Another study found that there was a sex-linked heritability to uricemia and gout development in a dwarf white leghorn strain (Cole et al., 1969).

Austic and Cole (1972) determined that the development of articular gout was associated with impaired renal clearance, as there was a decrease in renal tubular uric acid secretion by approximately 40% in birds with a predisposition to hyperuricemia and gout. Further studies confirmed the mechanism of a defect in renal tubular secretion of uric acid using dwarf white leghorn chickens that were selected for a high incidence of hyperuricaemia and articular gout (Zmuda and Quebbemann, 1975). Birds that demonstrated a 64% reduction in tubular excretion ratio developed articular gout (Zmuda and Quebbemann, 1975) with the site of this defect identified in the peritubular membrane.

A study by Guo et al. (2005) confirmed that excess dietary protein and calcium contributes to hyperuricaemia and development of visceral gout and kidney damage in growing laying hens. Additional studies have shown that in cases of hypervitaminosis D, or vitamin D toxicity, visceral gout can occur in macaw chicks (Takeshita et al., 1986). Vitamin D toxicity results in abnormally high calcium blood concentrations and which can be linked to gout conditions (Guo et al., 2005). Hypovitaminosis A can also be linked to gout conditions in birds. Crocodile hatchlings exposed to low vitamin A and high protein in the diet presented with hyperuricaemia and severe visceral gout which led to an increase in mortality (Ariel et al., 1997).

Wild bird populations have also been effected by articular and visceral gout. The Oriental white-backed vulture population has been in serious decline (< 95%) since the 1990's and has been recently placed on the critically endangered species list (Oaks et al., 2004). A contributing factor to the mortality of the vultures is the consumption of diclofenac, a common antibiotic used in livestock. In a study using contaminated carcass meat, researchers observed a high incidence of visceral gout in the vultures due to adverse effects on renal function by the drug (Oaks et al., 2004).

Treatments for avian gout include monitoring of dietary calcium, protein, and vitamin supplements. Allopurinol has also been used in cases of hyperuricaemia in Red-tailed Hawks (*Buteo jamaicensis*). However, there is an increase accumulation of xanthine in the blood, which precipitates in the renal tubules in a manner comparable to uric acid and can lead to nephropathy and possible renal failure (Ling et al., 1991). A study conducted by Lumeij and Redig (1992) found that allpurinol was toxic to red-tailed hawks at doses of 50 and 100 mg/kg body mass and exacerbated hyperuriceamia in the birds. Allopurinol was observed to cause vomiting and other toxic side effects (Lumeij et al., 1998) A follow-up to this study used a 25 mg/kg dose of allopurinol and determined that the dose was safe, but there were no changes in plasma uric acid, xanthine, hypoxanthine, allopurinol, and oxypurinol, making this a questionable treatment (Poffers et al., 2002). Thus under conditions which cause renal tubular secretion of uric acid to decline, there is an increase in the incidence of gout. High doses of allopurinol in birds are suggested to increase oxidative stress in treated birds, which increases mortality and therefore alternative treatments should be explored.

Conclusion

In conclusion, uric acid is vital to birds as an antioxidant defense mechanism. Birds have an elevated metabolism that should sustain increased amounts of oxidative damage over time and yet they live longer than mammalian counterparts of equal size. They achieve their longevity through several different mechanisms. Firstly, avian mitochondria are structurally unique from other species in that they have a highly efficient double packing of cristae which allows for greater performance of tissues such as flight muscle. Associated with this structure is a decreased release of ROS from the electron transport chain complexes. A proposed schematic of this mechanism can be observed in Figure 1. Secondly, the evolutionary loss of uricase can be linked to longer life spans as a consequence of increased plasma uric acid concentrations. The reason for the loss of uricase is still unclear though it is certainly links uric acid to antioxidant defense and has a role in longevity. Inexplicably, the enzyme that synthesizes uric acid, XOR, produces free radicals as a byproduct in the reaction with xanthine and hypoxanthine. Hyperuriceamia in birds results in failed renal transport, while allopurinol treatment is not free of severe adverse side effects. While there is a plethora of knowledge about uric acid, there is much to still learn about the regulation of XOR and the role of both uric acid and XOR in the antioxidant defense system.

Acknowledgment

This paper is submitted with the approval of the West Virginia Agricultural and Forestry Experimental Station (Scientific Article No. 3107).

References

Al-Seeni, A.E. 2009. Some biochemical studies on aldehyde oxidase and xanthine oxidase of agamid lizard uromastyx microlepis (Dhubb). *World Journal of Chemistry* 4(1): 45-51.

Alverez-Lario, B. and Macarron-Vicente, J. 2010. Uric acid and evolution. *Rheumatology*. 49: 2010-2015.

Ames, B., Cathcart, R., Schwiers, E., Hochstein, P. 1981. Uric acid provides an antioxidant defense in humans against oxidant and radical-caused aging and cancer: a hypothesis. *Proc. Natl. Acad. Sci*. 78(11): 6858-6862.

Angermuller, S., Bruder, G., Volkl, A., Wesch, H., Fahimi, H.D. 1987 . Localization of xanthine oxidase in crystalline cores of peroxisomes: a cytochemical and biochemical study. *European Journal of Cell Biology*. 47: 137-144.

Ariel, E., Ladds P.W., Buenviaje, G.N. 1997. Concurrent gout and suspected hypovitaminosis A in crocodile hatchlings. *Aust. Vet. J.* 4:247-249.

Aruoma, O. 1998. Free radicals, oxidative stress, and antioxidants in human health and disease. *JAOCS*. 75 (2): 199-211.

Austic, R. E. and Cole, R. K. 1972. Impaired renal clearance of uric acid in chickens having hyperuricemia and articular gout. *Am. J. Physiol.*, 223(3): 525-530.

Barja, G. 1998. Mitochondrial free radical production and aging in mammals and birds. *Annals of New York Academy of Sciences* 854(1): 224-238.

Barja, G. and Herrero, A. 1998. Localization at complex I and the mechanism of the higher free radical production if brain nonsynaptic mitochondria in the short-lived rat than in the longevous pigeon. *Journal of Bioenergetics and Biomembranes* 30(3):235-243.

Barja, G., Cadenas, S., Rojas, C., Perez-Campo, R., Lopez-Torres, M. 1994. Low mitochondrial free radical production per unit O_2 consumption can explain simultaneous presence of high longevity and high aerobic metabolic rate in birds.

Bataille, AM., Goldmeyer, J., Renfro, J. L. 2008. Avian renal proximal tubule epithelium urate secretion is mediated by Mrp4. *Am. J. Physiol. Integr. Comp. Physiol.* 295:2024-2033.

Beckman, K. and Ames, B. 1998. The free radical theory of aging matures. *Physiological Reviews* 78(2): 547-581.

Benboubetra, A., Gleeson, A., Harris, C.P.D., Kahn, J., Arrar, L., Brennand, D., Reid, J., Reckless, J.D., Harrison, R. 1997. Circulating anti-xanthine oxidoreductase antibodies in healthy human adults. *European Journal of Clinical Investigation* 27: 611-619.

Berry, C. and Hare, J. 2004. Xanthine oxidoreductase and cardiovascular disease: molecular mechanisms and pathophysiological implications. *Journal of Physiology* 555 (3): 589-606.

Braun, E. and W. Dantzler. 1997. Vertebrate renal system. In: *Handbook of Physiology. Comparative Physiology*. Bethesda, MD: *American Physiological Society*, sect.13, vol I, chapt. 8, pp 481-576.

Braun, E.J. and Dantzler, W.H. 1972. Function of mammalian-type and reptilian-type nephrons in kidney of desert quail. *Am. J. Physiol.* 222:617-629.

Brown, J., McClelland, G., Faure, P., Klaiman, J., Staples, J. 2009. Examining the mechanisms responsible for lower ROS rates in liver mitochondria from long-lived house sparrow (Passer domesticus), and big brown bat (Eptesicus fuscus) compared to the short-lived mouse (Mus musculus). *Mechanisms of Ageing and Development* 130: 467-476.

Bruder, G., Jarasch, E., Heid, H. 1984. High concentrations of antibodies to xanthine oxidase in human and animal sera: molecular characterization. *Journal of Clinical Investigation* 74: 783-794.

Cadenas, E. and Davies, K.J.A. 2000. Mitochondrial free radical generation, oxidative stress, and aging. *Free Radic. Biol. Med.* 29:222-230.

Carro, M.D, Falkenstein, E., Blemings, K.P., Klandorf, H. 2009. Determination of xanthine oxidoreductase activity in broilers: effect of pH and temperature of the assay and distribution in tissues. *Poult. Sci. Association* 88:2406-2414.

Carro, M.D., Falkenstein, E., Radke, W.J., Klandorf, H. 2009. Effects of allopurinol on uric acid concentrations, xanthine oxidoreductase activity, and oxidative stress in broiler chickens. *Comparative Biochemistry and Physiology*, Part C 151: 12-17.

Cazzaniga, G., Terao, M., Lo Schiavo, P., Galbiati, F., Segalla, F., Seldin, M.F., Garattino, E. 1994. Chromosomal mapping, isolation, and characterization of the mouse xanthine dehydrogenase gene. *Genomics* 23: 390-402.

Chen, Q., Vazquez, E., Mghaddas, S., Hoppel, C., Lesnefsky, E. 2003. Production of reactive oxygen species by mitochondria: central role of complex III. *The Journal of Biological Chemistry* 278(38): 36027-36031.

Chen, X.B., Samaraweera, L., Kyle, D.J., Orskov, E.R., Abeygunawardene, H. 1996. Urinary excretion of purine derivatives and tissue xanthine oxidase (EC 1.2.3.2) activity in buffalos(*Bubalis bubalis*) with special reference to differences between buffalo and *Bos taurus* cattle. *British Journal of Nutrition* 75: 397-407.

Cohen, A., Aberdroth, R., Hochstein, P. 1984. Inhibition of free radical-induced DNA damage by uric acid. *FEBS* 174 (1): 147-150.

Cohen, A., Klasing, K., Ricklefs, R. 2007. Measuring circulating antioxidants in wild birds. *Comparative Biochemistry and Physiology*. 147(B): 110-121.

Cole R.K., Austic, R. E., and Shane, S.M. 1969. Hereditary uriciemia and articular gout in chickens. *Poultry Sci.* 48: 1796.

Davies, K., Sevanian, A., Mukkassah-Kelly, S., Hochstein, P. 1986. Uric acid-iron complexes: a new aspect of the antioxidant functions of uric acid. *Biochem. J.* 235:747-754.

Della-Corte.E. and Stirpe, F. 1967. Regulation of xanthine dehydrogenase in chick liver: further experiments on the effects of inosine, actinomycin D, and other factors. *Biochemical Journal* 102: 520-524.

Devenyi, Z.J., Orchard, J.L., Powers, R.E. 1987. Xanthine oxidase activity in mouse pancreas: effects of caerulein-induced acute pancreatitis. *Biochemical and Biophysical Research Communications* 149(3): 841-845.

Dudas, P.L., Pelis, R.M., Braun, E. J., Renfro, J. L. 2005. Transepithelial urate transport by avian renal proximal tubule epithelium in primary culture. *J. Exp. Biol.* 208:4305-4315.

Fang, Y., Yank, S., Wu, G. 2002. Free radicals, antioxidants, and nutrition. *Nutrition* 18(10): 872-879.

Fhaolain, I.N. and Coughlan, M.P. 1978. Effects of allopurinol and oxypurinol on turkey liver xanthine dehydrogenase. *FEBS Letters* 90(2): 305-308.

Galbusera, C., Orth, P., Fedida, D., Spector, T. 2006. Superoxide radical production by allopurinol and xanthine oxidase. *Biochemical Pharmacology* 71: 1747-1752.

Garcia-Palmer, F. J., Pons, A., Alemany, M., Palou, A. 1985. Patterns of amino acid enzyme in domestic fowl breast and leg muscle during development. *Comparative Biochemistry and Physiology* 82B:143-146.

Guo, X., Huang, K., Tang, J.2005. Clinicopathology of gout in growing layers by high calcium and high protein diets. *British Poultry Science* 46(5): 641-646.

Halliwell, B. and Gutteridge, J.M.C. 1999. Free Radicals in Biology and Medicine third edition. Oxford University Press.

Hara, S., Mizukami, H., Mukai, T., Kurosaki, K., Kuriiwa, F. Endo, T. 2009. Involvement of extracellular ascorbate and iron in hydroxyl radical generation in rat striatum in carbon monoxide poisoning. *Toxicology* 264: 69-73.

Harris, C.M. and Massey V. 1997. The oxidative half-reaction of xanthine dehydrogenase with NAD; reaction kinetics and steady-state mechanism. *Journal of Biological Chemistry* 272: 28335-28341.

Harrison, R. 2002. Structure and function of xanthine oxidoreductase: where are we now? *Free Radical Biology and Medicine* 33(6): 774-797.

Hart, L.I., McGartoll, M.A., Chapman, R., Bray, R.C. 1970. The composition of milk xanthine oxidase. *Biochem J.* 116(5): 851-864.

Hille, R. and Anderson, R.F. 1991. Electron transfer in milk xanthine oxidase as studied by pulse radiolysis. *Journal of Biological Chemistry* 266: 5608-5615.

Hille, R. and Massey, V. 1981. Studies on the oxidative half- reaction of xanthine oxidase. *Journal of Biological Chemistry* 256: 9090-9095.

Hille, R. and Nishino, T. 1995. Xanthine oxidase and xanthine dehydrogenase. *FASEB Journal* 9: 995-1003.

Holmes,D.J. and Austad, S.N. 1995. The evolution of avian senescence patters; implications for understanding primary aging processes. *American Zooloogy* 35:307-317.

Hooper, D.C., Scott, G.S., Zborek, A., Miksheeva, T., Kean, R.B., Koprowski, H., Spitsin, S.V. 2000. Uric acid, a peroxynitrite scavenger, inhibits CNS inflammation, blood-CNS barrier permeability changes, and tissue damage in a mouse model of multiple sclerosis. *FASEB J.* 14: 691-698.

Hooper, D.C., Spitsin, S.V., Kean, R.B., Champion, J.M., Dickson, G.M., Chaudhry, I. 1998. Uric acid, a natural scavenger of peroxynitrite, in experimental allergic encephalomyelitis and multiple sclerosis. *Proc. Natl. Acad. Sci.* 95: 675-680.

Ichida, K., Matsumara, T., Sakuma, R., Hosoya, T., Nishino, T. 2001. Mutation of human molybdenum cofactor sulfurase gene responsible for classical xanthinuria type II. *Biochem. Biophys. Res. Commun.* 282: 1194-1200.

Ichikawa, M., Nishino, T., Nishino, T., Ichikawa, A. 1992. Subcellular localization of xanthine oxidase in rat hepatocytes. High resolution immunoelectron microscopic study combined with biochemical analysis. *Journal of Histochemistry and Cytochemistry* 40: 1097-1103.

Jarasch, E.D., Bruder, D., Heid, H.W. 1984. Significance of xanthine oxidase in capillary endothelial cells. *Acta Physiologica Scandinavica* 126: 39-46.

Jarasch, E.D., Grund, C., Bruder, D., Heid, H.W., Keenan, T.W., Franke, W.W. 1981. Localization of xanthine oxidase in mammary gland epithelium and capillary endothelium. *Cell* 25: 67-82.

Klandorf, H., Rathore, D.S., Iqbal, M., Shi, X., VanDyke, K. 2001. Accelerated tissue aging and increased oxidative stress in broiler chickens fed allopurinol. *Comp. Biochem. and Physiol.* Pt. C 129 (2): 93-104.

Kooij, A., Frederiks, W.M., Gossrau, R., Van Noorden, C.J.F. 1991. Localization of xanthine oxidoreductase activity using the tissue protectant polyvinyl alcohol and final electron acceptor tetranitro. *Journal of Histochemistry: Cytochemistry* 39:87-93.

Lane, N. 2005. Power, sex, suicide: mitochondria and the meaning of life. Oxford University Press, New York, pp-306-311.

Laverty, G. and Dantzler, W.H. 1983. Micropuncture study of urate transport by superficial nephrons in avian (*Sturnus vulgaris*) kidney. *Pflugers Arch.* 397: 232-236.

Ling, G.V., Ruby, A.L., Harrold, D.R., Johnson, D.L. 1991. Xanthine-containing calculi in dogs given allopurinol. *Journal of the American Veterinary Association*. 198:1935-1940.

Lumeij, J.T. and Redig, P.T. 1992. Hyperuriceamia and visceral gout induced by allopurinol in red-tailed hawks (*Buto jamaicensis*). *Proceedings VIII Tagung der Fachgruppe Geflugelkrankheiten* pp. 265-269.

Lumeij, J.T., Sprang, E.P.M., Redig, P.T. 1998. Further studies on allopurinol induced hyperuriceamia and visceral gout in red-tailed hawks (*Buto jamaicensis*). *Avian Pathology* 27:390-393.

Lyon E.S. and Garret, R.H. 1978. Regulation, purification, and properties of xanthine dehydrogenase in *Neurospora crassa*. *J. Biol. Chem*. 1978 253:2604-2614.

Machin, M., Simoyi, M., Blemings, K., Klandorf, H. 2004. Increased dietary protein elevates plasma uric acid and is associated with decreased oxidative stress in rapidly-growing broilers. *Comparative Biochemistry and Physiology Part B*. 137: 383-390.

Monnier,V.M., Sell, D.R., Ramanakoppa, H.N., Miyata, S. 1991. Mechanisms of damage mediated by the Maillard reaction in aging. *Gerontology* 37:152-165.

Moriwaki, Y., Yamamoto, T., Yamakita, J., Takahashi, S., Higashino, K. 1998. Comparative localization of aldehyde oxidase and xanthine oxidoreductase activity in rat tissues. *Histochemical Journal* 30: 69-74.

Munshi-South, J. and Wilkinson, G. 2009. Bats and birds: exceptional longevity despite high metabolic rates. *Ageing Research Reviews* 237: 1-8.

Murray, K.N., Watson, J.G., Chaykin, S. 1966. Catalysis of the direct transfer of oxygen from nicotinamide N-oxide to xanthine by xanthine oxidase. *Journal of Biological Chemistry* 241: 4798-4801.

Nishino, T., Nishino, T., Schopfer, L., Massey, V. 1989. The reactivity of chicken liver xanthine dehydrogenase with molecular oxygen. *Journal of Biological Chemistry* 264(5): 2518-2527.

Oaks, J. L., Gilbert, M., Virani, M.Z., Watson, R.T., Meteyer, C.U., Rideout, B.A., Shivaprasad, H.L., Ahmed, S., Chaudry, M.J.I., Arshad, M., Mahmood, S., All, A., Khan, A.A. 2004. Diclofenac residues as the cause of vulture population decline in Pakistan. *Nature* 427:630-633.

Oda, M., Satta, Y., Takenaka, O., Takahata, N. 2002. Loss of urate oxidase activity in hominoids and its evolutionary implications. *Mol. Biol. Evol.* 19 (5): 640-653.

Olson, J.S., Ballou, D.P., Palmer, G., Massey, V. 1974. The mechanism of action of xanthine oxidase. *J. Biol. Chem.* 249: 4363-4382.

Pacher, P., Nivorozhkin, A., Szabo, C. 2006. Therapeutic effects of xanthine oxidase inhibitors: renaissance half a century after the discovery of allopurinol. *Pharmacological Reviews* 58 (87): 87-114.

Pamplona, R., Portero-Otin, M., Sanz, A., Ayala, V., Vasileva, E., Barja, G. 2005. Protein and lipid oxidative damage and complex I content are lower in the brain of budgerigar and canaries than in mice. Relation to aging rate. *Age*. 27:267-280.

Parks, D.A., Granger, D.N. 1986. Xanthine oxidase: biochemistry, distribution, and physiology. *Acta Physiol. Scanda.* 548 (supplement): 87-99.

Pea, F. 2005. Pharmacology of drugs for hyperuricemia: mechanisms, kinetics, and interactions. Ronco, C. and Rodegheiro, F., Editors. Hyperuricemic syndromes: pathophysiology and therapy (Contributions to Nephrology). 147: 35-46. S. Karger Publications.

Peterson, D. W.., Hamilton, W. H. Lilyblade, A. L. 1971. Hereditary susceptibility to dietary induction of gout in selected lines of chickens. *J. Nutrition* 101:347-354.

Poffers, J., Lumeij, J.T., Timmermans-Sprang, E.P.M., Redig, P.T. 2002. Further studies on the use of allopurinol to reduce plasma uric acid concentrations in red-tailed hawks (*Buto jamaicensis)* hyperuraceamic model. *Avian Pathology*. 31:567-572.

Remy, C. and Westerfeld, W.W. 1951. The effect of diet on xanthine dehydrogenase in chicken tissues. *Journal of Biological Chemistry* 193(2): 659-667.

Rome, L. and Lindstedt, S. 1998. The quest for speed: muscles built for high-frequency contractions. *News Physiol. Sci.* 13:261-268.

Rosen,G.M., Pou,S., Ramos,C.L., Cohen,M.S., Britigan, B.E. 1995. Free radicals and phagocytic cells. The FASEB Journal 9(2): 200-209

Rouquette, M., Page, S., Bryant, R., Benboubetra, M., Stevens, C.R., Blake, D.R., Whish, W.J.D., Harrison, R., Tosh, D. 1998. Xanthine oxidoreductase is asymmetrically localized on outer surface of human endothelial and epithelial cells in culture. *FEBS Letters*. 426: 397-401.

Rowe, P., and Wyngaarden, J. 1966. The mechanism of dietary alterations in rat hepatic xanthine oxidase levels. *Journal of Biological Chemistry* 241(23): 5571-5576.

Saito, T. and Nishino, T. 1989. Differences in redox and kinetic properties between NAD-dependent and O_2-dependent types of rat liver xanthine dehydrogenase. *Journal of Biological Chemistry* 264: 10015-10022.

Sakamoto, N., Yamamoto, T., Moriwaki,Y., Teranishi, T., Toyoda, M., Onishi,Y., Kuroda, S., Sakaguchi, K., Fujisawa, T., Maeda, M., Hada, T. 2001. Identification of a new point mutation in the human xanthine dehydrogenase gene responsible for a case of classical type I xanthinuria. *Human Genetics* 108: 279-283.

Scholz, R.W. and Featherston, W.R. 1967. Effect of alterations in protein intake on liver xanthine dehydrogenase in the chick. *Journal of Nutrition* 95: 271-277.

Seaman, C., Moritz, J., Falkenstein, E., VanDyke, K., Casotti, G., Klandorf, H. 2008. Inosine ameliorates the effects of hemin-induced oxidative stress in broilers. *Comparative Biochemistry and Physiology*, Part A 151:670-675.

Shannon, J. A. 1983. The excretion of uric acid by the chicken. *J. Cell. Comp. Physiol.* 11:135-148.

Simoyi, M., VanDyke, K., Klandorf, H. 2002. Manipulation of plasma uric acid in broiler chicks and its effect on leukocyte oxidative activity. *Am. J. Physiol. Regulatory Integrative Comp. Phsyiol.* 282: 791-796.

Skinner K.A., Tan, S., Parks, D.A. 2001. Uric Acid Metabolism. Encyclopedia of Life Sciences. *Nature Publishing Group* / www.els.net. pp. 1-8.

Skinner KA, White CR, Patel R, Tan S, Barnes S, Kirk M, Darley-Usmar V, Parks DA. 1998. Nitrosation of uric acid by peroxynitrite. Formation of a vasoactive nitric oxide donor. *Journal of Biological Chemistry*, 273(38): 24491-7.

Slautterback, D. 1965. Mitochondria in cardiac muscle cells of the canary and some other birds. *The Journal of Cell Biology* 24:1-22.

Stewart, D.J., Holmes, W.N., Fletcher, G. 1969. The renal excretion of nitrogenous compounds by the duck (*Anas platyrhynchos*) maintained on freshwater and on hypertonic saline. *J. Exp. Biol.* 50:527-539.

Stinefelt,B., S.S. Leonard, K.P. Blemings, X.Shi, H. Klandorf. 2005. Free Radical Scavenging, DNA protection, and inhibition of lipid peroxidation mediated by uric acid. *Ann.Clin.Lab.Sci.* 35:37-45.

Strittmatter, C.F. 1965. Studies on avian xanthine dehydrogenases: properties and patterns of appearance during development. *Journal of Biological Chemistry* 240(6): 2557-2564.

Suarez, R.K., Lighton, J.R.B, Brown, G. S., Mathieu-Costello, O. 1991. Mitochondrial respiration in hummingbird flight muscles. *Proc. Natl. Acad. Sci.* 88:4870-4873.

Takeshita, K., Graham, D.L., Silverman, S. 1986. Hypervitaminosis D in baby macaws. *Proc. Assoc. Avian Vet. Miami* pp341-345.

Terada, L., Leff, J., Repine, J. 1990. Measurement of xanthine oxidase in biological tissues. *Methods in Enzymology* 186: 651-656.

Terao, M., Kurosaki, M., Zanotta, S., Garattini, E. The xanthine oxidoreductase gene: structure and regulation. *Biochemical Society Transactions* 25: 14170-14175.

Terzioglu, M. and Larson, N.G. 2007. Mitochondrial dysfunction in mammalian aging. *Mitochondrial Biology:New Perspectives*. Novartis Foundation. John Wiley and Sons, LTD. pp 197-213.

Thomas,C., Mackey, M.M., Diaz, A.A., Cox, D.P. 2009. Hydroxyl radical is produced via the Fenton reaction in submitochondrial particles under oxidative stress: implications for diseases associated with iron accumulation. *Redox Report* 14(3): 102-108.

Turrens, J. 2003. Mitochondrial formation of reactive oxygen species. *J. Physiol.* 552.2: 335-344.

VanDyke, K., VanDyke, C., Woodfork, K. 2002. *Luminescence Biotechnology Instruments and Applications*. CRC Press LLC.

Westerfeld, W.W., Richert, D.A., Hermans, A.C. 1962. Growth and liver xanthine dehydrogenase in chicks and poults fed casein or soy protein diet. *The Journal of Nutrition* 76: 475-482.

Xia, M., Dempski, R., Hille, R. 1999. The reductive half-reaction of xanthine oxidase- the reaction with aldehyde substrates and identification of the catalytically labile oxygen. *Journal of Biological Chemistry* 274: 3323-3330.

Xu, P., Hueksteadt, T.P., Hoidal, J.R. 1996. Molecular cloning and characterization of the human xanthine dehydrogenase gene. *Genomics* 34: 173-180.

Xu, P., Lavalee, P., Hoidal, J. R. 2000. Repressed expression of the human xanthine oxidoreductase gene. *J. Biol. Chem.* 275: 5918-5926.

Xu, P., Zhu, X.L., Huecksteadt, T.P., Brothman, A.R., Hoidal, J.R. 1994. Assignment of human xanthine dehydrogenase to chromosome 2p22. *Genomics* 23: 289-291.

Zmuda, M.J. and Quebbemann, A.J. 1975. Localization of renal tubular uric acid transport defect in gouty chickens. *Am. J. Physiol.* 229(3):820-825.

In: Uric Acid ISBN 978-1-62100-762-3
Editors: S. Castillo and E. Maldonado

Chapter II

Uric Acid in Multiple Sclerosis and Neurodegenerative Diseases

R. E. Gonsette
National Centre for Multiple Sclerosis, Melsbroek, Belgium

Abstract

Uric acid (UA) was long regarded as waste product. Since the early 1990s, the nonenzymatic antioxidant properties of UA have received increasing attention. It is now recognized that it accounts for over half of the antioxidant activity in human blood. Most of the neuroprotective activity of UA is related to its ability to scavenge peroxynitrite-derived free radicals before they can react with their targeted biological molecules.

Numerous observations and experimental data provide persuasive evidence for an altered metabolism of UA in diverse pathological states of the central nervous system (CNS) such as multiple sclerosis, optic neuritis, amyotrophic lateral sclerosis, Parkinson, Alzheimer, Huntington, Biswanger and variant Creutzfeld-Jakob diseases.

This wide involvement of UA is likely due to the fact that oxidative stress and excitotoxicity are the final interacting pathways leading to cell death, and that UA is a major antioxidant which also reduces glutamate toxicity.

The disturbances in UA metabolism are reflected by serum and cerebrospinal fluid (CSF) level changes. Most observations report lower

UA serum values in multiple sclerosis and neurodegenerative diseases. CSF and brain tissue UA levels are found lower in most neurodegenerative diseases compared with healthy people. By contrast, in multiple sclerosis and Biswanger disease, where the blood brain barrier is altered, UA concentrations seem higher than in normal brain.

Lower serum concentrations of UA may represent a primary, constitutive loss of protection against oxidative stress or a deficit secondary to UA consumption during oxidative radical scavenging. Higher concentrations of UA in CSF and brain may result from blood brain barrier leakage. Alternatively, they may reflect a rise in purine compounds degradation and consequently in their end product UA, due to an imbalance in ATP metabolism and energy state deficiency. In this hypothesis, UA would simply be an indirect marker of energy state imbalance.

Despite convincing experimental and clinical data indicating a potential neuroprotective role for UA in multiple sclerosis, a thoroughly conducted, placebo-controlled, double blind clinical trial maintaining an asymptomatic hyperuricaemia for 2 years did not provide any benefit on accumulation of disability in relapsing-progressing MS patients. The negative results of this trial supplementing a single antioxidative molecule, compared with the positive results of a recent clinical study activating the Nrf2-ARE pathway, suggest that activation of a global neuroprotective pathway is more effective than supplementation of one of its components alone.

Introduction

Uric acid (UA) is the terminal enzymatic product in the degradation of adenine and guanine-based metabolism. Present chiefly in the form of its monovalent anion (urate), it was long regarded as waste product. Roughly 20 million years ago, the urate oxydase (uricase) gene was progressively deactivated in human and great apes, concurrently with a stepwise decrease in the xanthine oxidase activity to allow adaptation to the loss of this important gene. The resulting inability to change UA in allantoïne has increased plasma UA levels by 10 times in humans compared with other mammals and is considered as an evolutionary advantage. . In 1981, Ames et al suggested that UA levels, which increased markedly during primate evolution, provide an antioxidant defence against oxidant- and free radical tissue damages [1]. Another possible advantage is that high plasma UA levels sustain serum salt levels and sufficiently high blood pressure in low salt environment [2]. A third benefit would be that UA targets purine receptors in the CNS and renders primates more mentally alert [3]. Of note that higher levels of UA are associated with a decreased risk of dementia and better cognitive function later in life [4].

Simultaneously, the ability to make ascorbic acid (AA), another potent nonenzymatic antioxidant, was lost [1]. In certain physiological conditions, reactions of UA with oxidants produce other radicals in particular urate radicals. This oxidant-antioxidant paradox might be explained by different effects of UA in various physicochemical circumstances or in different compartments of the human organism [5]. Of great relevance is the open question as to whether UA is beneficial or deleterious in the cardiovascular system which could possibly limit therapeutic use of UA. On the other hand, one of the sites where antioxidant effects of UA play a major role is the central nervous system (CNS) and a host of studies have demonstrated the neuroprotective activity of UA.

Oxidative Toxicity in Multiple Sclerosis

Peroxynitrite

Oxygen is essential for aerobic life but its metabolisms lead to the formation of harmful radical oxygen species (ROS). During species evolution, protective mechanisms against oxygen radicals have been progressively developed. The imbalance between ROS production and the natural antioxidant forces has been coined “oxidative stress” by Sies in 1985 [6].

During physiological conditions, basal levels of ROS are generated by all organisms. In mitochondria, a significant fraction of bimolecular oxygen (O2) is incompletely reduced and appears as ROS such as superoxide ($O2\bullet^-$), the hydroxyl radical (•OH) and hydroxyperoxide (H2O2). Those ROS are counterbalanced by natural enzymatic antioxidants (superoxide dismutase, catalase…) and non-enzymatic antioxidants (uric acid, ascorbic acid…). In pathological conditions elevated levels of ROS produced by inflammatory processes and mitochondria respiratory chain dysfunction overwhelm natural antioxidant defences and lead to oxidative stress.

The key effector molecule in oxidative stress is peroxynitrite (oxoperoxonitrate [−1]:$ONOO^-$). Peroxynitrite is generated *in vivo* by the combination of two ubiquitous free radicals: superoxide ($O2\bullet^-$) and •NO [7]. Excessive production of •NO is the driving force for peroxynitrite formation. Nitric oxide is an important biological messenger and plays a pivotal role in neurophysiology. However •NO can be neurotoxic as well as neuroprotective and it is the amount of •NO and the biological environment that determine its physiologic or pathophysiologic action. In the CNS, three canonical nitric oxide synthases (NOS) isoforms can generate •NO. Excessive production of •NO by activation of constitutive neuronal NOS (nNOS) is observed during mitochondrial respiratory chain dysfunction. Inducible NOS (iNOS) is located predominantly in macrophages and microglia and generates •NO in high levels and for extended periods during inflammatory reactions. Enhanced expression of the third isoform, constitutive endothelial NOS (eNOS) and subsequent local production of •NO; is associated with blood brain barrier (BBB) dysfunction. A fourth isoform has been recently identified, the mitochondrial NOS (mtNOS), a transcript of eNOS, producing reactive oxygen species (ROS) and representing a common pathophysiological etiology for many chronic diseases [8]. Peroxynitrite is rapidly protonated to peroxynitrous acid (hydrogen oxoperoxonitrate) that homolyzes to form nitrogen dioxide (•NO2) and the hydroxyl radical (•OH). For the most part, they recombine to form nitrate, a non-toxic product, but 30% leads to the formation of the highly toxic nitrite compound. In our biological environment, given the high concentration of the bicarbonate/carbon dioxide (CO2) pair, peroxynitrite reacts rapidly with CO2 to form •NO2 and carbonate radicals ($CO3\bullet^-$), two strong oxidants [9].

Peroxynitrite reacts with a bewildering number of molecules and remained a chemical curiosity for long. It has become to be accepted that peroxynitrite is the final, common toxic effector molecule responsible for oxidative stress damage in almost all pathological conditions including cardiac and vascular diseases, autoimmune local inflammation, brain and spinal cord injury, diabetes and diabetes complications and lastly neurodegenerative diseases and MS [10, 11]. Most of peroxynitrite pathomechanisms responsible for the protein and enzyme nitration are mediated via derived secondary oxidizing species. Highly toxic, peroxynitrite can nitrate and oxidize lipids, proteins, DNA and carbohydrates. In particular, peroxynitrite nitrates tyrosine residues, resulting in nitrotyrosine (NT) that can be identified immunohistochemically as a specific marker of peroxynitrite toxicity.

Peroxynitrite in Multiple Sclerosis

The presence of peroxynitrite in MS lesions as demonstrated by NT reactivity has been extensively investigated [12-14]. In acute lesions with intense perivascular and parenchymal infiltration, most NT-positive cells are mononuclear inflammatory cells. In chronic active lesions showing perivascular infiltrates and ongoing demyelination, NT-positive cells are predominantly lipid-laden macrophages, perivascular cells and ependymal cells from periventricular lesions. A prominent expression was noted in plaques with high inflammation. In contrast, in chronic silent lesions lacking an inflammatory component, NT-positive cells are absent [15]. In experimental allergic encephalomyelitis (EAE), peroxynitrite is formed very early, correlates with disease activity and cannot be detected during remissions and chronic, silent stages [16]. Both in MS and EAE, there is thus a clear correlation between inflammatory processes and peroxynitrite formation.

Interestingly, high levels of peroxiredoxin V, a natural enzymatic antioxidant, have been recently detected in normal appearing white matter from patients with MS, particularly in hypertrophic reactive astrocytes, not only in acute but also in chronic lesions [17]. This suggests that there is on-going oxidative stress in chronic lesions despite the absence of pathologically apparent inflammation. In contrast an elevated expression of myeloperoxidase in microglia was found in acute but not in chronic cortex demyelinating lesions [18]. The role of oxidative stress in MS is also supported by the correlation of Gd-enhancing lesions and of neurofilament damage markers with raised levels of nitric oxide metabolites in the cerebrospinal fluid (CSF) from MS patients [19, 20].

The predominant pathogenic role of peroxynitrite in EAE has been demonstrated after injection of a peroxynitrite catalyst specifically neutralizing peroxinitrite activity without affecting •NO mediated mechanisms [21]. Incidence and severity of clinical signs, inflammatory reactions, as well as NT immunoreactivity were markedly reduced. The prominent role of peroxynitrite is also reflected by the observation that mature oligodendrocytes are relatively resistant to direct •NO mediated toxicity but exquisitely sensitive to peroxynitrite-mediated injury [22].

In vivo damages of myelin and axons induced by peroxynitrite have been investigated in the rat [23]. Injection into the corpus callosum of a spontaneous donor of peroxynitrite produced vacuolization and destruction of myelin, similar to MS lesions. Amyloid precursor protein staining, a marker of axonal damage, was closely associated with demyelination and histopathology showed lesions characteristic of acute axonal lesions.

Due to their low antioxidant defences, neuronal cells are particularly vulnerable to oxidative toxicity. In EAE, peroxynitrite nitration of mitochondrial proteins is an early event, preceding infiltration of inflammatory cells and leading to several mitochondrial dysfunctions: respiratory chain depression, ATP synthesis reduction, membrane potential attenuation, imbalance in calcium homeostasis, reactive oxygen species (ROS) production, opening of permeability transition pores and DNA single strand breaks. Those peroxynitrite-induced mitochondrial impairments prime apoptosis of neuron and oligodendrocytes as well as axonal degeneration [24]. Tyrosine nitration by peroxynitrite is associated with inactivation of protein functions, especially of neurofilament-L proteins expressed in motor neurons and essential for their survival [25] as well as mitochondrial proteins, among which cytochrome C, Mn superoxide dismutase (SOD) and ATPase [26]. In MS, oxidative damage to mitochondrial DNA and mitochondrial enzymes has been observed in active chronic lesions [27]. Interestingly, in the pattern III subset of MS, mitochondrial respiratory dysfunction caused by oxidative stress results in pathological lesions similar to those observed in histotoxic hypoxia [28].

Astrocytes contain high concentrations of antioxidant enzymes and play a role in antioxidative processes [25]. However, inflammation induces iNOS expression in astrocytes leading to production of •NO that permeates astrocyte cell membrane and reacts with O2•_ to form peroxynitrite. The latter appears more deleterious to the neighbouring neurons than to the astrocytes themselves, but in response to extracellular peroxynitrite, astrocytes may become cytotoxic to motoneurons via peroxynitrite dependent mechanisms [29].

Like neurons, oligodendrocytes have low levels of antioxidant enzymes. Combined with a high iron content, this put them at increased risk for oxidative stress [30] and microglial toxicity to oligodendrocytes is mediated by peroxynitrite [31]. However, neurons are more sensitive than oligodendrocytes to oxidative toxicity and both are more sensitive to peroxynitrite than to NO toxicities. When cocultured with neurons, oligodendrocytes can imbue neurons with NO resistance through a protective factor that possibly could be heme-oxygenase-1 [32]. Importantly, several observations have demonstrated a maturation-dependent susceptibility of oligodendrocytes to free radical attacks [33, 34]. Oxidative toxicity could thus play a role not only in myelin destruction, but also in counteracting remyelination.

A strong expression of eNOS, a potential source of peroxynitrite, has been demonstrated in the intraparenchymal vascular endothelial cells of capillaries and venules of MS brains [35]. During their homing into CNS, overexpression of iNOS and •NO occurs in activated monocytes [36] and this may contribute to peroxynitrite formation inside endothelial cells and consequent damage of the BBB. Peroxynitrite also causes tight junction damage by altering zona occludens-1, f-actin and tight junction associated proteins [37] as well as other junctional protein expression [38]. It thus contributes to BBB dysfunction by disrupting both transcellular and paracellular paths [39]. Peroxynitrite also contributes to BBB leakage by enhancing expression of various endothelial adhesion molecules [40] but only in the presence of additional factors [41].

Lastly, free iron certainly plays a role in the pathogenesis of MS by catalyzing Fenton reactions that lead to oxidative damage. However, several therapeutic interventions targeting iron metabolism in EAE and MS patients remained inconclusive so far [42].

Uric Acid

Since the early 1990s, the specific antioxidant properties of UA have received increasing attention. Uric acid comprises 30–65% of the peroxyl radical-scavenging capacity of the plasma. On an equimolar basis, UA is 10 times as effective as ascorbate to scavenge singlet oxygen, H2O2, •OH, O2•⁻, •NO, •NO2 and CO3•⁻ [43]. Concentrations of UA are lower in the CNS than in other organs, and brain protein homogenates are more sensitive to peroxynitrite toxicity than heart protein homogenates [44]. Interestingly, it has been shown that ischemic preconditioning protection is partly mediated by natural antioxidant mobilisation, especially UA [45].

The efficiency of UA as neuroprotectant is definitely related to its ability to scavenge peroxynitrite-derived radicals before they can react with their targeted biological molecule. Indeed, the reaction of peroxynitrite with CO2 to form nitrosoperoxycarbonate which rapidly homolyzes to form NO2•⁻ and CO3•⁻, is 1000 times faster than the corresponding reaction with UA [46]. It has been demonstrated that NO2•⁻ and CO3•⁻ free radicals play a crucial role in peroxynitrite-mediated toxicity. Nitrogen dioxide preferentially reacts in environments such as cell membranes and hydrophobic protein domains, while CO3•⁻ can initiate lipid peroxidation, produce nitrated lipids and oxidize amino acids. Relevantly, UA concentrations around those present in human plasma inhibit completely tyrosine nitration *in vitro* [9].

Radical intermediates can be generated during the reactions of UA with peroxynitrite, notably the urate radical. The latter however is rapidly converted back to urate by ascorbate. There is thus a co-operative interaction between the two most important natural antioxidants, UA and ascorbate [47]. Experimentally, the antioxidant efficacy of UA in combination with ascorbate was found three times more important than that of UA alone. Ascorbate improves the ability of UA to act as an antioxidant by inhibiting radical intermediates generated by the interaction of UA with peroxynitrite [44]. Hooper and his group compared the protective effect of UA in acute EAE with that of a •NO scavenger(c-PTIO) and an iNOS inhibitor (D609). Only UA completely protected mice from EAE [48] and had a therapeutic effect when administered in animals with pre-existing disease.

The BBB is poorly permeable to UA but it is assumed that its compromised integrity in EAE facilitates the entrance of UA into the brain and that monocytes invading inflammatory lesions serve as a short-term reservoir of UA [49]. On the other hand, the BBB dysfunction associated with acute EAE is restored during UA administration [50]. The proposed mechanism is an inhibition of the production of TNF alpha by UA in neurovascular endothelial cells, a cytokine that upregulates ICAM-1 expression [51]. The antioxidant activity of UA was compared *in vitro* with that of ascorbic acid, cysteine and GSH, and UA proved to be the most effective scavenger [52].

It is generally accepted that UA has no effect on antigen presentation and recognition as well as on T cell priming and expansion [53]. However, the important role of UA in sterile inflammation has been recently reported. UA has been identified as one of the major danger signal (referred as damage-associated molecular patterns - DAMPs), released from injured cells to trigger sterile inflammation or to promote adaptive immune responses [54]. After cell death, nucleases rapidly degrade cell DNA and RNA. Liberated purines are converted into UA by xanthine oxidase leading to its accumulation. Physiological concentrations of UA are near-saturating and crystallization occurs easily. Monosodium urate crystals (MSU) drive the maturation of dendritic cells (DCs) and expression of costimulatory molecules CD80 and CD86. DCs prime the T cell inflammatory response and drive IL-1 production [55]. Importantly, the antioxidative activity of soluble UA balances the impact of MSU. In vivo, soluble UA restores a normal BBB permeability and hence reduces inflammation. The conversion of UA from a potent antioxidant into an inflammatory stimulant occurs only with large scale cell death causing the phase transition of soluble UA into MSU. The precise physiological conditions that regulate the balance between pro- and anti-inflammatory effects of UA in CNS pathological conditions as different as stroke and MS remain unclear.

Uric Acid and Multiple Sclerosis

In 1986, Honegger observed a major increase in UA levels in the spinal cord and serum from animals with EAE during attacks, followed by a reduction near normal values during recovery [56]. In contrast, no significant differences were found for other radical scavengers such as glutathione, cysteine, ascorbic acid and α-tocopherol [57]. To the best of our knowledge, only one publication concerned measurements of UA in MS brains and showed a marked increase in UA concentrations in plaques and peri-plaques compared with normal CNS tissue [58].

A few dosages of UA levels in serum and CSF of MS patients were performed using high-performance liquid chromatography (HPLC) and led to diverging results. In one publication, UA levels were reported lower both in serum and CSF [59] and unchanged in another study [60]. In serum, two investigations did not support alterations in UA metabolism [61, 62]. Interestingly, CSF UA levels were found increased in several observations [61, 63-65] in line with high UA levels observed in MS brains.

Most UA determinations in MS patients were assessed using commercially available enzymatic, colorimetric assays. Since the seminal publication of Hooper [66], a few publications excepted [67-70], decreased UA serum levels were consistently reported in patients with MS [71-82]. Notable is that serum UA levels were also found lower in clinically isolated symptoms [77], optic neuritis [83] and neuromyelitis optica [84].

Although the serum levels of UA were found to be low in MS, they were noted to be even lower during acute exacerbation versus remission periods [74, 80, 81, 85] and during relapsing versus secondary progressive stages [72, 77, 86]. Other correlations were less consistent. MS brain activity demonstrated by gadolinium-enhancing lesions inversely correlated with UA serum levels in some observations [72-74] but this was not confirmed later on [77, 84]. The same holds for inverse correlations of serum UA levels with disability and disease duration positive in some observations [73, 85] and absent in others [84].

There is cogent evidence that UA exerts potent antioxidant effect and hence a neuroprotective activity in various neuropathological conditions. First, the neuroprotective role of UA is experimentally substantiated by observations showing that, increased serum UA levels were found effective to reduce clinical and pathological signs in various experimental models: EAE [48], spinal cord injury [87], focal brain ischemia [88], experimental meningitis [89], lateral sclerosis amyotrophy [90] and Parkinson's disease (PD) [91, 92].

Experimentally, UA decreases the production and limits aggregation of the protease-resistant isoform of the prion protein which is thought to be the cause of neurodegeneration [93]. Second, increased serum UA levels appear to be associated with a lower risk of developing MS [48], Parkinson disease [94-99] and dementia [4]. Third, increased serum UA levels were reported during treatments with drugs whose efficacy is recognized in MS: glatiramer acetate [80, 100], high dose methylprednisolone [76, 80], IFNbs [76, 80, 101] and natalizumab [102].

The lower serum UA concentration in MS may represent a primary, constitutive loss of protection against oxidative stress [77] or a deficit secondary to UA consumption during oxidative radical scavenging [78]. In both cases, UA supplementation might be beneficial in MS patients.

Oral administration of UA does not increase serum UA levels because it is destroyed by gut microbial flora, but oral administration of inosine to MS patients increased UA levels both in serum and cerebrospinal fluid (CSF). [103]. Inosine was well tolerated and some evidence of benefit was suggested. In a recent trial, the possibility was tested that combined administration of interferon β (IFNβ), an anti-inflammatory drug, and inosine, an endogenous neuroprotective molecule, would be more effective than IFNβ alone on the accumulation of disability in RRMS patients [104]. In this multicentre, double-blind, placebo-controlled trial in 157 patients, an asymptomatic hyper-uricaemia was maintained for 2 years in the treated group. No difference was observed between the experimental and the control group concerning the number of patients with a neurological deterioration confirmed at three months, time to confirmed disability progression (Kaplan Meyer analysis), mean deterioration scale values (Expanded Disability Status Scale) [105] and time to first relapse.

Uric Acid and Neurodegenerative Diseases

Lower biological fluid UA levels have been documented in other auto-immune diseases such as Crohn's disease [106], myasthenia gravis and Guillain-Barré [107] as well as in neurodegenerative processes.

Lower serum UA concentrations were found in Huntington's disease [108], lateral sclerosis amyotrophy (ALS) [109, 110], Creutzfeld-Jakob's disease [93], Alzheimer's disease [111-113] and Parkinson's disease [97, 98, 114].

Lower CSF UA levels were observed in Huntington's disease [115], Creutzfeld-Jakob's disease [93], Alzheimer's disease [116] and Parkinson's disease [116, 117].

In addition to MS, higher CSF UA levels have been reported in Biswanger's disease supposedly due to alterations of the BBB [116].

Lower brain tissue UA concentrations were reported in Huntington's disease [115], Alzheimer's disease [118], Creutzfeld-Jakob's disease [93] and Parkinson's disease [117].

Lower brain tissue UA concentrations were reported in Huntington's disease [115], Alzheimer's disease [118], Parkinson's disease [117, 119] and Creutzfeld-Jakob's disease [93].

Correlations between higher UA serum levels and slower disease progression have been documented in Huntington's disease [120] and ALS [110]. Correlations between cognitive functions and serum UA levels have been recently demonstrated. Higher serum UA levels are associated with a decreased risk of dementia and better function later in life [121] and UA transporter gene SLC2A9 polymorphysms are associated with increased performance on memory-related tasks [122]. In patients with mild cognitive impairment, baseline serum UA levels do not predict conversion to Alzheimer's disease but are associated with a reduced rate of cognitive decline [123]. Experimental data suggest that administration of UA might prevent or attenuate decline in cognitive functions in patients with Alzheimer's disease [124].

The most detailed correlations between UA and neurodegenerative disorders have been performed in Parkinson's disease. However, it is not clear yet if they apply to both sexes as several observations were limited to men. Serum UA levels were found consistently lower compared with healthy controls [97, 98, 114]. Baseline low UA serum levels are associated with a decreased risk of developing the disease [95, 99]. A significant reduction in the incidence is observed among individual with a history of gout [96, 125, 126]. The rate of disability progression is lower in patients with high serum UA levels [94] and they have a lower percentage of striatal cell loss as demonstrated by a radiographic marker for the presynaptic dopamine transporter [127]. Both serum and CSF UA levels measured at baseline are inversely related to clinical progression [128]. The rate of disability progression is lower in patients with high serum UA levels [94] and they have a lower percentage of striatal cell loss as demonstrated by a radiographic marker for the presynaptic dopamine transporter [127]. Additionally, it has been suggested that UA transporter gene (SLC2A9) polymorphisms influence age at onset [129]. A clinical trial is in progress to evaluate the potential benefit of inosine administration on Parkinson's disease evolution (http://clinicaltrial.gov, NCT00833690).

Conclusion

There is now mounting evidence that UA plays an essential role in neurodegenerative processes including MS. Neurodegeneration results from a pathogenic cascade including multiple and interacting pathomechanisms such as oxidative stress, excitotoxicity, mitochondriopathy and ion channel dysfunction leading to cell apoptosis or necrosis.

There is compelling evidence that UA exerts a dual neuroprotective role. First, it is the major component of low molecular weight endogenous antioxidants and is a potent scavenger of peroxynitrite mediated oxidative toxicity. It also activates redox-sensitive glutamate transport elements such as excitatory amino-acid transporter 1 and reduces excitotoxicity. Second, UA produced by purines liberated during cell death, acts as a major endogenous danger signal promoting adaptive immune responses. A host of clinical and experimental observations have shown that UA concentrations are altered in biological fluids and brain tissue in neurodegenerative diseases but the question arises as to whether and how UA metabolism alterations can interfere with their development and progression.

The results concerning UA serum levels in MS are sometimes conflicting but emerging findings suggest that they are decreased in most patients especially during clinical and radiological disease activity. Data in neurodegenerative diseases are more consistent and it has come to be accepted that decreases in UA serum levels are statistically significant. The reduction observed in MS and degenerative diseases compared with controls is relatively modest (10-15%) and one may question their clinical significance given the 60% difference between the upper and lower limits of the reference range of normal UA serum levels. It seems unlikely that UA serum levels changes may serve as a reliable marker of disease activity and response to therapy.

Observations concerning UA concentrations in CSF and brain tissues are more informative. UA levels are consistently decreased in all neurodegenerative diseases with the exception of MS and Biswanger's disease where they are markedly increased. In the latter, increased UA CSF concentrations are clearly associated with BBB leakage but information concerning UA levels in brain tissue is lacking so far. In MS brains, the highest UA concentrations are found in plaques and wane with increasing distance suggesting a blood origin. It is well established that BBB alterations exist in MS mainly during acute disease activity. On the other hand, elevated UA levels in the CNS from MS patients might reflect decreased brain ATP synthesis causing cell energy state imbalance and subsequent outflow of ATP catabolites including UA precursors [65]. In this hypothesis, UA would be an indirect marker of energy state imbalance.

Clinical correlations with UA serum levels concerning the risk of developing the disease or the progression of disability appear more reliable in neurodegenerative diseases than in MS. Intriguingly, in Parkinson's disease most correlations were observed only in men. The question is whether those sex-specific differences are related to serum UA level imbalance between men and women or to the disease itself. Given that non steroidal anti-inflammatory drugs in contrast protect against Parkinson's disease only in women [130], it seems that the mere differences in serum UA levels between genders cannot explain sex-specific effects and that Parkinson's disease pathophysiology might be heterogeneous.

Considerable circumstantial evidence has accumulated that UA levels are reduced in biological fluids and brain tissue of neurodegenerative diseases and supports the notion of a deregulation of defences against oxidative stress. Whether this reflects an intrinsically reduced UA reserve or a consumption of UA as a scavenger of ROS and whether lower levels UA levels are a cause or a consequence of the disease remains an open question.

Both experimental and clinical data strongly suggest that increasing UA levels would afford neuroprotection in neurodegenerative diseases. In MS patients, an asymptomatic hyperuricaemia maintained for 2 years did not provide any additional benefit on accumulation of disability and cerebral atrophy in RRMS patients. A first explanation might be that UA dosage was too low. In animals, basal serum UA levels are definitely lower than in humans. Large amounts of antioxidant are required to protect effectively against EAE and they induce a marked increase in serum and CNS UA levels [131]. For safety reasons, in clinical trials, serum UA levels must be maintained within the limits of asymptomatic hyperuricaemia. The important differences in UA metabolism between mammals and humans possibly explain why effective animal models are found poorly predictive of clinical benefits.

Direct LMWA, including UA, are consistently up-regulated in MS brains [132]. One may thus wonder if antioxidant neuroprotection can be further harnessed or whether it is already maximally stimulated. In that case, boosting further antioxidant production will be ineffective.

Another concern is the most effective stage in a specific pathogenic pathway to interfere with. UA does not react directly with peroxynitrite but scavenge its peroxynitrite-derived radical species. Blocking peroxynitrite production upstream might be more effective.

Lastly and most importantly, there is a growing appreciation that endogenous neuroprotection is the net result of several complex and intermingled mechanisms [133].

UA is a member of the direct LMWA and there is growing awareness that modulating an individual component of a neuroprotective pathway will likely yield a partial benefit, if any. A derivative of the fumeric acid (BG0012) activates the indirect (phase2) LMWA pathway via the "nuclear factor erythroid 2-related factor 2" (Nrf2) and induces the production of several enzymatic and non-enzymatic antioxidants. Notably, the activation of this complex pathway reduced MRI active lesions in a phase II clinical trial [134, 135] suggesting that activation of a global pathway is more effective than supplementation of one of its components alone.

Further studies are necessary to understand the precise molecular mechanisms underlying neuroprotective pathways and their complex interconnections. It would also be of central interest to monitor activated pathways to identify their respective roles at a certain point of time and their specific activation according to pathomechanism stages and microenvironment status.

References

[1] Ames BN, Cathcart R, Schwiers E, Hochstein P. Uric acid provides an antioxidant defense in humans against oxidant- and radical-caused aging and cancer: a hypothesis. Proc. Natl. Acad. Sci. USA 1981; 78: 6858-6862.

[2] Watanabe S, Kang DH, Feng L, Nakagawa T, Kanellis J, Lan H, Mazzali M, Johnson RJ. Uric acid, hominoid evolution, and the pathogenesis of salt-sensitivity. *Hypertension* 2002: 40: 355-360.

[3] Sofaer JA, Emery AE. Genes for super-intelligence? *J Med Genet* 1981; 18: 410-413.

[4] Euser SM, Hofman A, Westendorp RG, Breteler MM. Serum uric acid and cognitive function and dementia. *Brain* 2009; 132: 377-382.

[5] Sautin YY, Johnson RJ. Uric acid: the oxidant-antioxidant paradox. *Nucleosides Nucleotides Nucleic Acids* 2008; 27: 608-619.

[6] Sies H. Oxidative stress: Introductory remarks. In: Sies H, editor. Oxidative stress. London, Academic Press, 1985, 1-7.

[7] Beckman JS, Beckman TW, Chen J, Marshall PA, Freeman BA. Apparent hydroxyl radical production by peroxynitrite: implications for endothelial injury from nitric oxide and superoxide. *Proc. Natl. Acad. Sci. USA* 1990; 87: 1620-1624.

[8] Finocchietto PV, Franco MC, Holod S, Gonzalez AS, Converso DP, Arciuch VG, Serra MP, Poderoso JJ, Carreras MC. Mitochondrial nitric oxide synthase: a masterpiece of metabolic adaptation, cell growth, transformation, and death. *Exp. Biol. Med.* 2009; 234: 1020-1028.

[9] Augusto O, Bonini MG, Amanso AM, Linares E, Santos CC, De Menezes SL. Nitrogen dioxide and carbonate radical anion: two emerging radicals in biology. *Free Radic. Biol. Med.* 2002; 32: 841-859.

[10] Pacher P, Beckman JS, Liaudet L. Nitric oxide and peroxynitrite in health and disease. *Physiol. Rev.* 2007; 87: 315-424.

[11] Sayre LM, Perry G, Smith MA. Oxidative stress and neurotoxicity. *Chem. Res. Toxicol.* 2008; 21: 172-188.

[12] Cross AH, Manning PT, Keeling R M, Schmidt RE, Misko TP. Peroxynitrite formation within the central nervous system in active multiple sclerosis. *J. Neuroimmunol.* 1998; 88: 45-56.

[13] Oleszak EL, Zaczynska E, Bhattacharjee M, Butunoi C, Legido A, Katsetos CD. Inducible nitric oxide synthase and nitrotyrosine are found in monocytes/macrophages and/or astrocytes in acute, but not in chronic, multiple sclerosis. *Clin. Diagn Lab. Immunol.* 1998; 5: 438-445.

[14] Liu JS, Zhao ML, Brosnan CF, Lee SC. Expression of inducible nitric oxide synthase and nitrotyrosine in multiple sclerosis lesions. *Am. J. Pathol.* 2001; 158: 2057-2066.

[15] Hill KE, Zollinger LV, Watt HE, Carlson NG, Rose JW. Inducible nitric oxide synthase in chronic active multiple sclerosis plaques: distribution, cellular expression and association with myelin damage. *J. Neuroimmunol.* 2004; 151: 171-179.

[16] Van der Veen RC, Hinton DR, Incardonna F, Hofman FM. Extensive peroxynitrite activity during progressive stages of central nervous system inflammation. *J. Neuroimmunol.* 1997; 77: 1-7.

[17] Holley JE, Newcombe J, Winyard PG, Gutowski NJ. Peroxiredoxin V in multiple sclerosis lesions: predominant expression by astrocytes. *Mult. Scler.* 2007; 13: 955-961.

[18] Gray E, Thomas TL, Betmouni S, Scolding N, Love S. Elevated activity and microglial expression of myeloperoxidase in demyelinated cerebral cortex in multiple sclerosis. *Brain Pathol.* 2008; 18: 86-95.

[19] Rejdak K, Eikelenboom MJ, Petzold A, Thompson EJ, Stelmasiak Z, Lazeron RH, et al. CSF nitric oxide metabolites are associated with activity and progression of multiple sclerosis. *Neurology* 2004; 63: 1439-1445.

[20] Rejdak K, Petzold A, Stelmasiak Z, Giovannoni G. Cerebrospinal fluid brain specific proteins in relation to nitric oxide metabolites during relapse of multiple sclerosis. *Mult. Scler.* 2008; 14: 59-66.

[21] Cross AH, San M, Stern MK, Keeling RM, Salvemini D, Misko TP. A catalyst of peroxynitrite decomposition inhibits murine experimental autoimmune encephalomyelitis. *J. Neuroimmunol.* 2000; 107: 21-28.

[22] Jack CS, Kuhlmann T, Antel JP. Differential susceptibility of human adult oligodendrocytes to injury mediated by nitric oxide and peroxynitrite. *Neurology* 2004; 62 (suppl 5): A117 (abstract).

[23] Touil T, Deloire-Grassin MS, Vital C, Petry KG, Brochet B. In vivo damage of CNS myelin and axons induced by peroxynitrite. *Neuroreport* 2001; 12: 3637-3644.

[24] Qi X, Lewin AS, Sun L, Hauswirth WW, Guy J. Mitochondrial protein nitration primes neurodegeneration in experimental autoimmune encephalomyelitis. *J. Biol. Chem.* 2006; 281: 31950-31965.

[25] Strong M, Sopper M, He BP. In vitro reactive nitrating species toxicity in dissociated spinal motor neurons from NFL (-/-) and hNFL (+/+) transgenic mice. *Amyotroph Lateral Scler. Other Motor. Neuron. Disord* 2003; 4: 81-89.

[26] Radi R. Nitric oxide, oxidants, and protein tyrosine nitration. *Proc. Natl. Acad. Sci. USA* 2004; 101: 4003-4008.

[27] Lu F, Selak M, O'Connor J, Croul S, Lorenzana C, Butunoi C, Kalman B. Oxidative damage to mitochondrial DNA and activity of mitochondrial enzymes in chronic active lesions of multiple sclerosis. *J. Neurol. Sci.* 2000; 177: 95-103.

[28] Aboul-Enein F, Lassmann H. Mitochondrial damage and histotoxic hypoxia: a pathway of tissue injury in inflammatory brain disease? *Acta Neuropathol.* 2005; 109: 49-55.

[29] Cassina P, Peluffo H, Pehar H, Martinez-Palma L, Ressia A, Beckman JS, Estévez AG, Barbeito L. Peroxynitrite triggers a phenotypic transformation in spinal cord astrocytes that induces motor neuron apoptosis. *J. Neurosci. Res.* 2002; 67: 21-25.

[30] Smith KJ, Kapoor R, Felts PA. Demyelination: the role of reactive oxygen and nitrogen species. *Brain Pathol.* 1999; 9: 69-92.

[31] Li J, Baud O, Vartanian T, Volpe JJ, Rosenberg PA. Peroxynitrite generated by inducible nitric oxide synthase and NADPH oxidase mediates microglial toxicity to oligodendrocytes. *Proc. Natl. Acad. Sci. USA* 2005; 102: 9936-9941.

[32] Bishop A, Hobbs KG, Eguchi A, Jeffrey S, Smallwood L, Pennie C, Anderson J, Estévez AG. Differential sensitivity of oligodendrocytes and motor neurons to reactive nitrogen species: implications for multiple sclerosis. *J. Neurochem.* 2009; 109: 93-104.

[33] Bernardo A, Greco A, Levi G, Minghetti L. Differential lipid peroxidation, Mn superoxide, and bcl-2 expression contribute to the maturation-dependent vulnerability of oligodendrocytes to oxidative stress. *J. Neuropathol. Exp. Neurol.* 2003; 62: 509-519.

[34] Baud O, Haynes RF, Wang H, Folkerth RD, Li J, Volpe JJ, Rosenberg PA. Developmental up-regulation of MnSOD in rat oligodendrocytes confers protection against oxidative injury. *Eur. J. Neurosci.* 2004; 20: 29-40.

[35] Broholm H, Andersen B, Wanscher B, Frederiksen JL, Rubin I, Pakkenberg B, Larsson HB, Lauritzen M. Nitric oxide synthase expression and enzymatic activity in multiple sclerosis. *Acta Neurol. Scand.* 2004; 109: 261-269.

[36] Sarchielli P, Orlacchio A, Vicinanza F, Pelliccioli GP, Tognoloni M, Saccardi C, Gallai V. Cytokine secretion and nitric oxide production by mononuclear cells of patients with multiple sclerosis. *J. Neuroimmunol.* 1997; 80: 76-86.

[37] Mazzon E, De Sarro A, Caputi AP, Cuzzocrea S. Role of tight junction derangement in the endothelial dysfunction elicited by exogenous and endogenous peroxynitrite and poly(ADP-ribose) synthetase. *Shock* 2002; 18: 434-439.

[38] Zhang Y, Zhao S, Gu Y, Lewis DF, Alexander JS, Wang Y. Effects of peroxynitrite and superoxide radicals on endothelial monolayer permeability: potential role of peroxynitrite in preeclampsia. *J. Soc. Gynecol. Investig.* 2005; 12: 586-92.

[39] Kirk J, Plumb J, Mirakhur M, McQuaid S. Tight junctional abnormality in multiple sclerosis white matter affects all calibres of vessel and is associated with blood-brain barrier leakage and active demyelination. *J. Pathol.* 2003: 201: 319-27.

[40] Zouki C, Zhang SL, Chan JS, Filep JG. Peroxynitrite induces integrin-dependent adhesion of human neutrophils to endothelial cells via activation of the Raf-1/MEK/Erk pathway. *FASEB J.* 2001: 15: 25-27.

[41] Bolton C, Wood EG, Scott GS, Flower RJ. A comparative evaluation of the response to peroxynitrite by a brain endothelial cell line and control of the effects by drug targeting. *Cell Mol. Neurobiol.* 2009; 29: 707-717.

[42] Levine SM, Chakrabarty A. The role of iron in the pathogenesis of experimental allergic encephalomyelitis and multiple sclerosis. *Ann. NY Acad. Sci.* 2004; 1012: 252-266.

[43] Becker BF. Towards the physiological function of uric acid. *Free Radic. Biol. Med.* 1993; 14: 615-631.

[44] Kuzkaya N, Weissmann N, Harrison DG, Dikalov S. Interactions of peroxynitrite with uric acid in the presence of ascorbate and thiols: implications for uncoupling endothelial nitric oxide synthase. *Biochem. Pharmacol.* 2005; 70: 343-354.

[45] Glantz L, Avramovich A, Trembovler V, Gurvitz V, Kohen R, Eidelman LA, et al. Ischemic preconditioning increases antioxidants in the brain and peripheral organs after cerebral ischemia. *Exp. Neurol.* 2005; 192: 117-124.

[46] Squadrito GL, Cueto R, Splenser AE, Valavanidis A, Zhang H, Uppu RM, Pryor WA. Reaction of uric acid with peroxynitrite and implications for the mechanism of neuroprotection by uric acid. *Arch. Biochem. Biophys.* 2000; 376: 333-337.

[47] Bowman GL, Shannon J, Frei B, Kaye JA, Quinn JF. Uric acid as a CNS antioxidant. *J. Alzheimers Dis.* 2010; 19: 1331-1336.

[48] Hooper DC, Bagasra O, Marini JC, Zborek A, Ohnishi ST, Kean R Champion JM, Sarker AB, Bobroski L, Farber JL, Akaike T, Maeda H, Koprowski H. Prevention of experimental allergic encephalomyelitis by targeting nitric oxide and peroxynitrite: implications for the treatment of multiple sclerosis. *Proc. Natl. Acad. Sci. USA* 1997; 94: 2528-2533.

[49] Spitsin SV, Scott GS, Kean RB, Mikheeva T, Hooper DC. Protection of myelin basic protein immunized mice from free-radical mediated inflammatory cell invasion of the central nervous system by the natural peroxynitrite scavenger uric acid. *Neurosci. Lett.* 2000; 292: 137-41.

[50] Hooper DC, Scott GS, Zborek A, Mikheeva T, Kean RB, Koprowski H, Spitsin SV. Uric acid, a peroxynitrite scavenger, inhibits CNS inflammation, blood-CNS barrier permeability changes, and tissue damage in a mouse model of multiple sclerosis. *FASEB J.* 2000; 14: 691-698.

[51] Scott GS, Kean RB, Fabis MJ, Mikheeva T, Brimer CM, Phares TW Spitsin SV, Hooper DC. ICAM-1 upregulation in the spinal cords of PLSJL mice with experimental allergic encephalomyelitis is dependent upon TNF-alpha production triggered by the loss of blood-brain barrier integrity. *J. Neuroimmunol.* 2004; 155: 32-42.
[52] Spitsin SV, Scott GS, Mikheeva T, Zborek A, Kean RB, Brimer CM, Koprowski H, Hooper DC. Comparison of uric acid and ascorbic acid in protection against EAE. *Free Radic. Biol. Med.* 2002; 33: 1363-1371.
[53] Kean RB, Spitsin SV, Mikheeva T, Scott GS, Hooper DC. The peroxynitrite scavenger uric acid prevents inflammatory cell invasion into the central nervous system in experimental allergic encephalomyelitis through maintenance of blood-central nervous system barrier integrity. *J. Immunol.* 2000; 165: 6511-6518.
[54] Shi Y, Evans JE, Rock KL. Molecular identification of a danger signal that alerts the immune system to dying cells. *Nature* 2003; 425: 516-521.
[55] Kono H, Chen CJ, Ontiveros F, Rock KL. Uric acid promotes an acute inflammatory response to sterile cell death in mice. *J. Clin. Invest.* 2010; 120: 1939-1949.
[56] Honegger CG, Krenger W, Langemann H. Increased concentrations of uric acid in the spinal cord of rats with chronic relapsing experimental allergic encephalomyelitis. *Neurosci. Lett.* 1986; 69: 109-114.
[57] Honegger CG, Krenger W, Langemann H. Measurement of free radical scavengers in the spinal cord of rats with experimental autoimmune encephalomyelitis. *Neurosci. Lett.* 1989; 98: 327-332.
[58] Langemann H, Kabiersch A, Newcombe J. Measurement of low-molecular-weight antioxidants, uric acid, tyrosine and tryptophan in plaques and white matter from patients with multiple sclerosis. *Eur. Neurol.* 1992; 32: 248-252.
[59] Reiber H, Ruff M, Uhr M. Ascorbate concentration in human cerebrospinal fluid (CSF) and serum. Intrathecal accumulation and CSF flow rate. *Clin. Chim. Acta* 1993; 217: 163-173.
[60] Kastenbauer S, Kieseier BC, Becker BF. No evidence of increased oxidative degradation of urate to allantoin in the CSF and serum of patients with multiple sclerosis. *J. Neurol.* 2005; 252: 611-612.
[61] Karg E, Klivényi P, Németh I, Bencsik K, Pintér S, Vécsei L. Nonenzymatic antioxidants of blood in multiple sclerosis. *J. Neurol.* 1999; 246: 533-539.
[62] Becker BF, Kastenbauer S, Ködel U, Kiesl D, Pfister HW. Urate oxidation in CSF and blood of patients with inflammatory disorders of

the nervous system. *Nucleosides Nucleotides Nucleic Acids* 2004; 23: 1201-1204.

[63] Kuracka L, Kalnovicová T, Líska B, Turcáni P. HPLC method for measurement of purine nucleotide degradation products in cerebrospinal fluid. *Clin. Chem.* 1996; 42:756-760.

[64] Stover JF, Lowitzsch K, Kempski OS. Cerebrospinal fluid hypoxanthine, xanthine and uric acid levels may reflect glutamate-mediated excitotoxicity in different neurological diseases. *Neurosci. Lett.* 1997; 238: 25-28.

[65] Amorini AM, Petzold A, Tavazzi B, Eikelenboom J, Keir G, Belli A, Giovannoni G, Di Pietro V, Polman C, D'Urso S, Vagnozzi R, Uitdehaag B, Lazzarino G. Increase of uric acid and purine compounds in biological fluids of multiple sclerosis patients. *Clin. Biochem.* 2009; 42: 1001-1006.

[66] Hooper DC, Spitsin S, Kean RB, Champion JM, Dickson GM, Chaudhry I, Koprowski H. Uric acid, a natural scavenger of peroxynitrite, in experimental allergic encephalomyelitis and multiple sclerosis. *Proc. Natl. Acad. Sci. USA* 1998; 95: 675-680.

[67] Kanabrocki EL, Ryan MD, Hermida RC, Ayala DE, Scott GS, Murray D, Bremner WF, Third JL, Johnson MC, Foley S, Van Cauteren J, Shah F, Shirazi P, Nemchausky BA, Hooper DC. Altered circadian relationship between serum nitric oxide, carbon dioxide, and uric acid in multiple sclerosis. *Chronobiol. Int.* 2004; 21: 739-758.

[68] Ramsaransing GS, Heersema DJ, De Keyser J. Serum uric acid, dehydroepiandrosterone sulphate, and apolipoprotein E genotype in benign vs progressive multiple sclerosis. *Eur. J. Neurol.* 2005; 12: 514-518.

[69] Mostert JP, Ramsaransing GS, Heersema DJ, Heerings M, Wilczak N, De Keyser J. Serum uric acid levels and leukocyte nitric oxide production in multiple sclerosis patients outside relapses. *J. Neurol. Sci.* 2005; 231: 41-44.

[70] Salemi G, Gueli MC, Vitale F, Battaglieri F, Guglielmini E, Ragonese P, Trentacosti A, Massenti MF, Savettieri G, Bono A. Blood lipids, homocysteine, stress factors, and vitamins in clinically stable multiple sclerosis patients. *Lipids Health Dis.* 2010; 9: 19.

[71] Spitsin S, Hooper DC, Mikheeva T, Koprowski H. Uric acid levels in patients with multiple sclerosis: analysis in mono- and dizygotic twins. *Mult. Scler.* 2001; 7: 165-166.

[72] Drulović J, Dujmović I, Stojsavljević N, Mesaros S, Andjelković S, Miljković D, Perić V, Dragutinović G, Marinković J, Lević Z, Mostarica Stojković. Uric acid levels in sera from patients with multiple sclerosis. *J. Neurol.* 2001; 248: 121-126.

[73] Sotgiu S, Pugliatti M, Sanna A, Sotgiu A, Fois ML, Arru G, Rosati G. Serum uric acid and multiple sclerosis. *Neurol. Sci.* 2002; 23: 183-188.

[74] Toncev G, Milicic B, Toncev S, Samardzic G. Serum uric acid levels in multiple sclerosis patients correlate with activity of disease and blood-brain barrier dysfunction. *Eur. J. Neurol.* 2002; 9: 221-226.

[75] Galboiz Y, Miller A. Immunological indicators of disease activity and prognosis in multiple sclerosis. *Curr. Opin. Neurol.* 2002; 15: 233-237.

[76] Deretzi G, Pelidou SH, Zacharakis G, Kyritsis AP. Serum levels of uric acid in patients with multiple sclerosis: a biological marker in clinical course and treatment of MS. *Mult. Scler.* 2003; 9(suppl 1): S100, P412.

[77] Rentzos M, Nikolaou C, Anagnostouli M, Rombos A, Tsakanikas K, Economou M, Dimitrakopoulos A, Karouli M, Vassilopoulos D. Serum uric acid and multiple sclerosis. *Clin. Neurol. Neurosurg.* 2006; 108: 527-531.

[78] Koch M, Ramsaransing GS, Arutjunyan AV, Stepanov M, Teelken A, Heersema DJ, De Keyser J. Oxidative stress in serum and peripheral blood leukocytes in patients with different disease courses of multiple sclerosis. *J. Neurol.* 2006; 253: 483-487.

[79] Peng J, Dicker B, Du W, Tang F, Nguyen P, Geiger T, Wong FS, Wen L. Converting antigen-specific diabetogenic CD4 and CD8 T cells to TGF-beta producing non-pathogenic regulatory cells following FoxP3 transduction. *J. Autoimmun.* 2007; 28: 188-200.

[80] Guerrero AL, Martín-Polo J, Laherrán E, Gutiérrez F, Iglesias F, Tejero MA, Rodríguez-Gallego M, Alcázar C. Variation of serum uric acid levels in multiple sclerosis during relapses and immunomodulatory treatment. *Eur. J. Neurol.* 2008; 15: 394-397.

[81] Tsakiri A, Tsiantoulas D, Frederiksen J. Serum uric acid levels are decreased in patients with relapsing-remitting multiple sclerosis, in particular during relapses. *Mult. Scler.* 2008; 14(suppl 1):S289, P888.

[82] Zamani A, Rezaei A, Khaeir F, Hooper DC. Serum and cerebrospinal fluid uric acid levels in multiple sclerosis patients. *Clin. Neurol. Neurosurg.* 2008; 110: 642-643.

[83] Knapp CM, Constantinescu CS, Tan JH, McLean R, Cherryman GR, Gottlob I. Serum uric acid levels in optic neuritis. *Mult. Scler.* 2004; 10: 278-280.

[84] Peng F, Zhong X, Deng X, Qiu W, Wu A, Long Y, Hu X, Li Q, Jiang Y, Dai Y. Serum uric acid levels and neuromyelitis optica. *J. Neurol.* 2010; 257: 1021-1026.

[85] Guerrero AL, Gutiérrez F, Iglesias F, Martín-Polo J, Merino S, Martín-Serradilla JI, Laherrán E, Tejero MA. Serum uric acid levels in multiple sclerosis patients inversely correlate with disability. *Neurol. Sci.* 2011; 32: 347-350.

[86] Dujmovic I, Pekmezovic T, Obrenovic R, Nikolić A, Spasic M, Mostarica Stojkovic M, Drulovic J. Cerebrospinal fluid and serum uric acid levels in patients with multiple sclerosis. *Clin. Chem. Lab. Med.* 2009; 47: 848-853.

[87] Scott GS, Cuzzocrea S, Genovese T, Koprowski H, Hooper DC. Uric acid protects against secondary damage after spinal cord injury. *Proc. Natl. Acad. Sci. USA* 2005; 102: 3483-3488.

[88] Yu ZF, Bruce-Keller AJ, Goodman Y, Mattson MP. Uric acid protects neurons against excitotoxic and metabolic insults in cell culture, and against focal ischemic brain injury in vivo. *J. Neurosci. Res.* 1998; 53: 613-625.

[89] Kastenbauer S, Koedel U, Becker BF, Pfister HW. Experimental meningitis in the rat: protection by uric acid at human physiological blood concentrations. *Eur. J. Pharmacol.* 2001; 425: 149-152.

[90] Guermonprez L, Ducrocq C, Gaudry-Talarmain YM. Inhibition of acetylcholine synthesis and tyrosine nitration induced by peroxynitrite are differentially prevented by antioxidants. *Mol. Pharmacol.* 2001; 60: 838-846.

[91] Anderson RF, Harris TA. Dopamine and uric acid act as antioxidants in the repair of DNA radicals: implications in Parkinson's disease. *Free Radic. Res.* 2003; 37: 1131-1136.

[92] Duan W, Ladenheim B, Cutler RG, Kruman II, Cadet JL, Mattson MP. Dietary folate deficiency and elevated homocysteine levels endanger dopaminergic neurons in models of Parkinson's disease. *J. Neurochem.* 2002; 80: 101-110.

[93] Lekishvili T, Sassoon J, Thompsett AR, Green A, Ironside JW, Brown DR. BSE and vCJD cause disturbance to uric acid levels. *Exp. Neurol.* 2004; 190: 233-244.

[94] Davis JW, Grandinetti A, Waslien CI, Ross GW, White LR, Morens DM. Observations on serum uric acid levels and the risk of idiopathic Parkinson's disease. *Am. J. Epidemiol.* 1996; 144: 480-484.

[95] De Lau LM, Koudstaal PJ, Hofman A, Breteler MM. Serum uric acid levels and the risk of Parkinson disease. *Ann. Neurol.* 2005; 58: 797-800.
[96] Alonso A, Rodríguez LA, Logroscino G, Hernán MA. Gout and risk of Parkinson disease: a prospective study. *Neurology* 2007; 69: 1696-1700.
[97] Annanmaki T, Muuronen A, Murros K. Low plasma uric acid level in Parkinson's disease. *Mov. Disord.* 2007; 22: 1133-1137.
[98] Weisskopf MG, O'Reilly E, Chen H, Schwarzschild MA, Ascherio A. Plasma urate and risk of Parkinson's disease. *Am. J. Epidemiol.* 2007; 166: 561-567.
[99] Gao X, Chen H, Choi HK, Curhan G, Schwarzschild MA, Ascherio A. Diet, urate, and Parkinson's disease risk in men. *Am. J. Epidemiol.* 2008; 167: 831-838.
[100] Constantinescu CS, Freitag P, Kappos L. Increase in serum levels of uric acid, an endogenous antioxidant, under treatment with glatiramer acetate for multiple sclerosis. *Mult. Scler.* 2000; 6: 378-381.
[101] Toncev G, Drakulic M, Knezevic Z. Treatment with interferon beta 1b (Betaferon) and serum uric acid levels: two year follow-up. *Mult. Scler.* 2007; 13(suppl 2): S90, P305.
[102] Handouk Y, Angeleri VA, Danni M, De Riso S, Provinciali L. Increase of serum uric acid levels in multiple sclerosis during treatment with natalizumab. *Mult. Scler.* 2008; 14(suppl 1): S281, P888.
[103] Koprowski H, Spitsin SV, Hooper DC. Prospects for the treatment of multiple sclerosis by raising serum levels of uric acid, a scavenger of peroxynitrite. *Ann. Neurol.* 2001; 49: 139.
[104] Gonsette RE, Sindic C, D'hooghe MB, De Deyn PP, Medaer R, Michotte A, Seeldrayers P, Guillaume D; ASIIMS study group. Boosting endogenous neuroprotection in multiple sclerosis: the ASsociation of Inosine and Interferon beta in relapsing- remitting Multiple Sclerosis (ASIIMS) trial. *Mult. Scler.* 2010; 16: 455-462.
[105] Kurtzke JF. Rating neurologic impairment in multiple sclerosis: an expanded disability status scale (EDSS). *Neurology* 1983; 33: 1444-1452.
[106] Rezaie A, Ghorbani F, Eshghtork A, Zamani MJ, Dehghan G, Taghavi B, Nikfar S, Mohammadirad A, Daryani NE, Abdollahi M. Alterations in salivary antioxidants, nitric oxide, and transforming growth factor-beta 1 in relation to disease activity in Crohn's disease patients. *Ann. NY Acad. Sci.* 2006; 1091: 110-122.

[107] Peng F, Zhang B, Zhong X, Li J, Xu G, Hu X, Qiu W, Pei Z. Serum uric acid levels of patients with multiple sclerosis and other neurological diseases. *Mult. Scler.* 2008; 14: 188-196.

[108] Insarova NG, Korshunova TS, Mzhel'skaia TI, Borisova TV. Metabolic disorders in Huntington's chorea. *Zh. Nevropatol. Psikhiatr. Im. S S Korsakova* 1978; 78: 489-495.

[109] Sohmiya M, Tanaka M, Suzuki Y, Tanino Y, Okamoto K, Yamamoto Y. An increase of oxidized coenzyme Q-10 occurs in the plasma of sporadic ALS patients. *J. Neurol. Sci.* 2005; 228: 49-53.

[110] Keizman D, Ish-Shalom M, Berliner S, Maimon N, Vered Y, Artamonov I, Tsehori J, Nefussy B, Drory VE. Low uric acid levels in serum of patients with ALS: further evidence for oxidative stress? *J. Neurol. Sci.* 2009; 285: 95-99.

[111] Rinaldi P, Polidori MC, Metastasio A, Mariani E, Mattioli P, Cherubini A, Catani M, Cecchetti R, Senin U, Mecocci P. Plasma antioxidants are similarly depleted in mild cognitive impairment and in Alzheimer's disease. *Neurobiol. Aging* 2003; 24: 915-919.

[112] Polidori MC, Mattioli P, Aldred S, Cecchetti R, Stahl W, Griffiths H, Senin U, Sies H, Mecocci P. Plasma antioxidant status, immunoglobulin g oxidation and lipid peroxidation in demented patients: relevance to Alzheimer disease and vascular dementia. *Dement Geriatr Cogn. Disord* 2004; 18: 265-270.

[113] Kim TS, Pae CU, Yoon SJ, Jang WY, Lee NJ, Kim JJ, Lee SJ, Lee C, Paik IH, Lee CU. Decreased plasma antioxidants in patients with Alzheimer's disease. *Int. J. Geriatr Psychiatry* 2006; 21: 344-348.

[114] Larumbe Ilundáin R, Ferrer Valls JV, Viñes Rueda JJ, Guerrero D, Fraile P. Case-control study of markers of oxidative stress and metabolism of blood iron in Parkinson's disease. *Rev. Esp. Salud Publica* 2001; 75: 43-53.

[115] Beal MF, Matson WR, Storey E, Milbury P, Ryan EA, Ogawa T, Bird ED. Kynurenic acid concentrations are reduced in Huntington's disease cerebral cortex. *J. Neurol. Sci.* 1992; 108: 80-87.

[116] Tohgi H, Abe T, Takahashi S, Kikuchi T. The urate and xanthine concentrations in the cerebrospinal fluid in patients with vascular dementia of the Binswanger type, Alzheimer type dementia, and Parkinson's disease. *J. Neural. Transm. Park Dis. Dement Sect.* 1993; 6: 119-126.

[117] Church WH, Ward VL. Uric acid is reduced in the substantia nigra in Parkinson's disease: effect on dopamine oxidation. *Brain Res. Bull* 1994; 33: 419-425.

[118] Hensley K, Maidt ML, Yu Z, Sang H, Markesbery WR, Floyd RA. Electrochemical analysis of protein nitrotyrosine and dityrosine in the Alzheimer brain indicates region-specific accumulation. *J. Neurosci.* 1998; 18: 8126-8132.

[119] Fitzmaurice PS, Ang L, Guttman M, Rajput AH, Furukawa Y, Kish SJ. Nigral glutathione deficiency is not specific for idiopathic Parkinson's disease. *Mov. Disord.* 2003; 18: 969-976.

[120] Auinger P, Kieburtz K, McDermott MP. The relationship between uric acid levels and Huntington's disease progression. *Mov. Disord.* 2010; 25: 224-228.

[121] Euser SM, van Bemmel T, Schram MT, Gussekloo J, Hofman A, Westendorp RG, Breteler MM. The effect of age on the association between blood pressure and cognitive function later in life. *J. Am. Geriatr. Soc.* 2009; 57: 1232-1237.

[122] Houlihan LM, Wyatt ND, Harris SE, Hayward C, Gow AJ, Marioni RE, Strachan MW, Price JF, Starr JM, Wright AF, Deary IJ. Variation in the uric acid transporter gene (SLC2A9) and memory performance. *Hum. Mol. Genet.* 2010; 19: 2321-2330.

[123] Irizarry MC, Raman R, Schwarzschild MA, Becerra LM, Thomas RG, Peterson RC, Ascherio A, Aisen PS. Plasma urate and progression of mild cognitive impairment. *Neurodegener Dis.* 2009; 6: 23-28.

[124] Waugh WH. Inhibition of iron-catalyzed oxidations by attainable uric acid and ascorbic acid levels: therapeutic implications for Alzheimer's disease and late cognitive impairment. *Gerontology* 2008; 54: 238-243.

[125] De Vera M, Rahman MM, Rankin J, Kopec J, Gao X, Choi H. Gout and the risk of Parkinson's disease: a cohort study. *Arthritis. Rheum.* 2008; 59: 1549-1554.

[126] Alonso A, Sovell KA. Gout, hyperuricemia, and Parkinson's disease: a protective effect? *Curr. Rheumatol. Rep.* 2010; 12: 149-155.

[127] Schwarzschild MA, Schwid SR, Marek K, Watts A, Lang AE, Oakes D, Shoulson I, Ascherio A; Parkinson Study Group PRECEPT Investigators, Hyson C, Gorbold E, Rudolph A, Kieburtz K, Fahn S, Gauger L, Goetz C, Seibyl J, Forrest M, Ondrasik J. Serum urate as a predictor of clinical and radiographic progression in Parkinson disease. *Arch. Neurol.* 2008; 65: 716-723.

[128] Ascherio A, LeWitt PA, Xu K, Eberly S, Watts A, Matson WR, Marras C, Kieburtz K, Rudolph A, Bogdanov MB, Schwid SR, Tennis M, Tanner CM, Beal MF, Lang AE, Oakes D, Fahn S, Shoulson I, Schwarzschild MA; Parkinson Study Group DATATOP Investigators. Urate as a predictor of the rate of clinical decline in Parkinson disease. *Arch. Neurol.* 2009; 66: 1460-1468.

[129] Facheris MF, Hicks AA, Minelli C, Hagenah JM, Kostic V, Campbell S, Hayward C, Volpato CB, Pattaro C, Vitart V, Wright A, Campbell H, Klein C, Pramstaller PP. Variation in the uric acid transporter gene SLC2A9 and its association with AAO of Parkinson's disease. *J. Mol. Neurosci.* 2011; 43: 246-250.

[130] Wahner AD, Bronstein JM, Bordelon YM, Ritz B. Nonsteroidal anti-inflammatory drugs may protect against Parkinson disease. *Neurology* 2007; 69: 1836-1842.

[131] Scott GS, Spitsin SV, Kean RB, Mikheeva T, Koprowski H, Hooper DC. Therapeutic intervention in experimental allergic encephalomyelitis by administration of uric acid precursors. *Proc. Natl. Acad. Sci. USA* 2002; 99: 16303-16308.

[132] van Horssen J, Schreibelt G, Drexhage J, Hazes T, Dijkstra CD, van der Valk P, de Vries HE. Severe oxidative damage in multiple sclerosis lesions coincides with enhanced antioxidant enzyme expression. *Free Radic. Biol. Med.* 2008; 45: 1729-1737.

[133] Gonsette RE. Endogenous neuroprotection in multiple sclerosis. *Acta Neurol. Belg.* 2010; 110: 26-35.

[134] Kappos L, Gold R, Miller DH, Macmanus DG, Havrdova E, Limmroth V, Polman CH, Schmierer K, Yousry TA, Yang M, Eraksoy M, Meluzinova E, Rektor I, Dawson KT, Sandrock AW, O'Neill GN; BG-12 Phase IIb Study Investigators. Efficacy and safety of oral fumarate in patients with relapsing-remitting multiple sclerosis: a multicentre, randomised, double-blind, placebo-controlled phase IIb study. *Lancet* 2008; 372: 1463-1472.

[135] Gold R, Linker RA, Stangel M. Fumaric acid and its esters: An emerging treatment for multiple sclerosis with antioxidative mechanism of action. *Clin. Immunol.* 2011; [Epub ahead of print].

In: Uric Acid
Editors: S. Castillo and E. Maldonado
ISBN 978-1-62100-762-3

Chapter III

Role of Uric Acid in Metabolic Syndrome

Andréa Name Colado Simão[1] *and Isaias Dichi* [2]
[1] Department of Pathology, Clinical Analysis, and Toxicology, University of Londrina, Paraná, Brazil
[2] Department of Internal Medicine, University of Londrina, Paraná, Brazil

Abstract

Metabolic syndrome (MS) comprises pathological conditions that include insulin resistance, arterial hypertension, obesity and dyslipidemia; associated abnormalities include inflammation and endothelial dysfunction. Uric acid increase is considered an important risk factor for the development of cardiovascular disease favoring oxidative stress and endothelial dysfunction, thus being involved in MS pathophisiology. There is supporting evidence that uric acid may have a pathogenic role in the metabolic syndrome. Insulin has a physiologic action on renal tubules, causing a reduction in uric acid clearance, what could explain the

[1] Andréa Name Colado Simão, PhD, Address: Department of Pathology, Clinical Analysis and Toxicology. Rua Robert Koch no 60 Bairro Cervejaria, University of Londrina. Londrina, Paraná, Brazil. CEP: 86038-440, Telephone: (55) 43 3371 2331, E-mail: deianame@gmail.com , FAX: (55) 43 3371 2323
[2] Corresponding author: Isaias Dichi, MD, PhD, Address: Department of Internal Medicine. Rua Robert Koch n. 60 Bairro Cervejaria, University of Londrina. Londrina, Paraná, Brazil. CEP: 86038-440, Telephone: (55) 43 3371 2332 ,E-mail: dichi@sercomtel.com.br, FAX: (55) 43 3371 5100

higher uric acid levels found in MS. It was hypothesized a causal role of uric acid in fructose-induced metabolic syndrome showing that uric acid dose dependently blocked acethylcholine mediated arterial dilatation, suggesting that uric acid can impair endothelial function. In addition, it was verified that allopurinol, a xanthine oxidase inhibitor that lowers serum uric acid, was able to decrease systolic blood pressure, improve insulin sensitivity, and normalize triacylglycerol levels in fructose-induced metabolic syndrome. Moreover, uric acid can contribute to oxidative stress present in MS. Uric acid may trigger the reactive oxygen substances (ROS) generation through various mechanisms, for instance, activating the NADPH oxidase system. This statement was demonstrated in adypocites. ROS increase give raise to peroxinitrite ($ONOO^-$) by reaction with nitric oxide (NO) leading to protein nitrosylation, lipid peroxidation and NO• reduction altering endothelial function. Furthermore, uric acid has been shown to reduce NO bioavailability in various cell types via mechanisms involving redox control and also activating arginase and depleting NO. Uric acid can also form free radicals in various reactions, including peroxynitrite whose products are responsible for the amplification of lipid oxidation. However, it has also an important role in the antioxidant defense system. Uric acid is an important antioxidant, being responsible for 60% of the scavenging activity of the free radicals in human plasma. Uric acid reduces organic peroxyl radicals (ROO•) into hydroperoxide (ROOH), blockading its degradation to low molecular weight aldehydes. There is a positive correlation between uric acid levels and total antioxidant capacity. Therefore, uric acid seems to have a double role in oxidative stress measurements. Uric acid involvement in oxidative and nitroactive stress is very complex because its antioxidant/prooxidant capacity and probably this balance are concentration and pH dependent. Although uric acid may have a protective effect due to its antioxidant properties, it is clear that the dominant effect of uric acid in MS is deleterious. Long-term studies to verify the consequences of decreasing uric acid concentration below current recommendations in asymptomatic patients are needed.

Introduction

The importance of hyperuricemia and the clustering phenomenon of the metabolic syndrome (MS) were first described by Kylin in 1923 when he described the clustering of three clinical syndromes: hypertension, hyper-glycemia, and hyperuricemia. Seven decades after the clustering phenomenon was reported by Kylin, Zavaroni and Reaven (1993) suggested that hyper-uricemia should be added to the cluster of metabolic and hemodynamic abnormalities associated with insulin resistance and/or hyperinsulinemia of MS. Markedly increased levels of uric acid (> 6.2 mg/dL or 370 uM) are known to cause gout and nephrolithiasis, but more importantly have been associated with increased risk for the development of cardiovascular disease, particularly hypertension and MS.

Uric acid is a purine metabolite that in most mammals is degraded by the hepatic enzyme uricase to allantoin [Mazzali et al., 2001].The absence of the enzyme uricase has been considered an evolutionary stage as urate may have evolved as a compensatory mechanism in higher primates that have lost the capacity to generate other antioxidants *in vivo* [George and Stuthers, 2009]. In turn, xanthine oxidase is a rate-limiting enzyme which primary role is the conversion of hypoxanthine to xanthine and xanthine to urate. Despite the efficient mechanisms developed to excrete urate, serum acid uric can be readily increased by diet, particularly meat and seafood rich in purine, alcohol and fructose, whereas low-fat dairy products have the opposite effect and purine-rich vegetables, such as beans, lentils, peas, spinach, etc, have no detrimental effects on uric acid concentration [Choi et al., 2004; Sánchez-Lozada et al., 2006]. Twenty years ago, Facchini et al. (1991) had suggested the mechanisms by which insulin action could enhance uric acid concentration. Since then, besides a consequence of metabolic disturbances, hyperuricemia has been reported as a strong independent predictor of the development of hypertension in longitudinal studies in adults [Sundström et al., 2005] and children [Alper et al., 2005] and even a predictor of metabolic syndrome [Choi and Ford, 2007]. Hence, the classical view of uric acid as a simple and innocent bystander has been challenged and has turned into a more complex understanding of its dual role, as consequence of hypertension and metabolic syndrome, but also as a cause of hypertension, and likely implicated in the etiology of metabolic syndrome. There is a growing body of evidence to support the role of hypertension as the link between hyperuricemia and metabolic syndrome [Lin et al., 2004; Khosla et al., 2005].

Uric acid has also a dual role in prooxidant/antioxidant state. Uric acid possesses free-radical-scavenging properties and is the most abundant antioxidant in human plasma (Ames et al., 1981) being responsible for 60% of total antioxidant capacity. Of note, in conditions in which hyperuricemia may occur, as, for instance, metabolic syndrome, total antioxidant status may be increased due to enhanced uric acid concentration [Simão et al., 2008]. Urate may serve as a primary antioxidant because it can remove singlet oxygen and radicals as effective as vitamin C in humans [Choi et al., 2004]. In addition, uric acid also stimulates the expression of extracellular superoxide dismutase which may confer additional antioxidant protection [Sánchez-Lozada et al., 2006]. It is noteworthy that strategies to improve antioxidant protection using uric acid were suggested in the treatment of patients with multiple sclerosis [Koprovski et al., 2001]. On the other hand, uric acid may also act as a prooxidant under conditions of oxidative stress. The two major systems generating vascular oxidative stress are the xanthine oxidase and the nicotinamide adenine dinucleotide phosphate (NADPH) oxidase pathways [George and Stuthers, 2009]. Besides being the final product of xanthine oxidase pathway, uric acid may even activate the NADP oxidase system [Sautin et al., 2007].

Therefore, the aim of the present review is to contribute to the understanding of the physiopathological mechanisms underlying the dual role of uric acid as cause and consequence in metabolic syndrome as well as its dual role in prooxidant/antioxidant sate.

Uric Acid as a Predictor of the Development of Hypertension and Metabolic Syndrome

The knowledge that hypertension is strongly associated with hyperuricemia has many decades. Serum uric acid levels are elevated in hypertension and are present in 25% of untreated hypertensive subjects, 50% of subjects taking diuretics, and more than 75% of patients with malignant hypertension [Cannon et al., 1966].

Several reports have pointed out that even after adjusted for confounding factors, hyperuricemia can predict the development of coronary artery disease, heart failure, stroke, renal disease, and type 1 diabetes mellitus [Feig et al., 2008; Hovind et al, 2009]. Similarly, hypertension, obesity, hyperinsulinemia, type 2 diabetes mellitus, and metabolic syndrome can be predicted by hyperuricemia [Choi and Ford, 2007; Feig et al., 2008]. Even with normal range of serum acid concentration, the risk of metabolic syndrome was found to be elevated in proportion to uric acid concentration (Yoo et al., 2005). There is a growing body of evidence that hypertension may be the factor that links hyperuricemia and metabolic syndrome [Lin et al., 2004; Khosla et al., 2005; Mené and Punzo, 2008; Feig et al., 2008; Gagliardi et al., 2009]. First, hyper-uricemia is common in primary hypertension, whereas it is not observed in secondary hypertension. Second, some human studies have reported that allopurinol, a xanthine oxidase inhibitor, reduced significantly hypertension in a similar magnitude of others antihypertensive agents. Third, fructose intake has been suggested to induce hyperuricemia, and subsequently hypertension, and metabolic syndrome both in experimental and human studies [Kanellis and Kang, 2005; Choi et al., 2008]. Nakagawa et al. (2006) hypothesized a causal role of uric acid in fructose-induced metabolic syndrome showing that uric acid dose dependently blocked acethylcholine mediated arterial dilatation, suggesting that uric acid can impair endothelial function. In addition, they verified that allopurinol, a xanthine oxidase inhibitor that lowers serum uric acid, was able to decrease systolic blood pressure, improve insulin sensitivity, and normalize triacylglycerol levels in fructose-induced metabolic syndrome. Fourth, in mammals, only men and apes do not have the hepatic enzyme uricase, which converts uric acid to alantoin. In a rat model of hyperuricemia induced by an uricase inhibitor, hypertension occurred after several weeks and decreased values were observed after treatment with a xanthine oxidase inhibitor, a uricosuric agent, by supplementing with L-arginine, a nitric oxide synthase (NOS) substrate, or blocking angiotensin II formation with enalapril. Hence, it was suggested that both angiotensin II and NO are involved in hypertension induced by uric acid [Mazzali et al, 2001]. In this model, endothelial dysfunction mediated by decreased nitric oxide concentrations was implicated, as it was also verified in human studies [Mercuro et al., 2004; Ho et al., 2010]. In turn, glucose uptake in skeletal muscle depends on nitric oxide release from endothelial cells. As, in this system, nitric oxide release is reduced, derangement in carboidrate metabolism occurs [Nakagawa et al, 2006]. Several studies in animal models support the role of uric acid as a predictor of metabolic syndrome and report that reduction in uric acid concentrations can prevent or reverse features in metabolic syndrome (Nakagawa et al., 2006; Sánchez-Lozada et al., 2008). Furthermore, metabolic syndrome has been described in mice lacking endothelial nitric oxide synthase [Cook et al., 2003]. Fifth, clinical trials have demonstrated that uric acid concentration predicts renal dysfunction, which is associated with the development of hypertension (Tsoulis et al., 2006).

Richard Johnson and colleagues [2002a, 2002b, 2005a, 2005b] suggested that hypertension induced by hyperuricemia would be mediated by two mechanisms. The first mechanism would result from uric acid-induced renal vasoconstriction mediated by endothelial dysfunction with reduced nitric oxide levels and by activation of the renin-angiotensin system. This hypertension type is salt-resistant and responds to lowering of uric acid. After that, when hyperuricemia causes progressive renal microvascular disease, hypertension becomes salt-driven, renal dependent, and independent of uric acid levels. This hypothesis justifies several findings. First, the relationship between hyperuricemia and hypertension verified in epidemiological studies is stronger for younger subjects than older subjects; renal evolvement in older subjects may explain this observation. Second, in experimental studies, when increased uric acid concentration cause renal injury, animals develop salt-sensitive hypertension, regardless of the level of uric acid. The mechanism of the persistent salt sensitivity is thought to be due to renal ischemia leading to activation of renal renin-angiotensin system, vasoconstriction, and increased sodium reabsorption. Third, some forms of secondary hypertension may not be cured by treating the underlying cause if the kidneys show vascular changes. Therefore, it seems that maintaining a lower uric acid would be more effective at prevention rather than lowering uric acid in the treatment of hypertension because once intra-renal vascular disease develops, hypertension is then driven by renal disease [Alper et al., 2005]. Hence, thiazide diuretic agents would be inappropriate for the treatment of the initial phase of salt-resistant hypertension and, by increasing uric acid and rennin may actually worsen the underlying cause of hypertension [Johnson et al., 2005b].

On the other hand, some authors observed that the strongest association in predicting metabolic syndrome features was verified between uric acid and abdominal obesity [Onat et al., 2006; Ford et al., 2007]. The reasons why abdominal obesity may be the link between uric acid and metabolic syndrome seem weaker than the abovementioned reasons which pointed out hypertension as the more probable link. The strongest argument against this likelihood is the finding that only 5.9% of subjects with normal body mass index and uric acid concentration less than 6.0 mg/dL had metabolic syndrome, whereas 59% of subjects with normal body mass index and uric acid above 10 mg/dL had evidence of metabolic syndrome [Choi and Ford, 2007]. Nevertheless, an interesting finding which favors abdominal obesity as the link factor between uric acid and metabolic syndrome is that uric acid and leptin, a pro inflammatory cytokine secreted by adipocytes, tend to rise together and leptin may affect renal uric acid absorption [Choi et al., 2004]. Leptin levels are elevated and associated with insulin resistance in MS and early T2DM. It is possible that leptin is a regulator of serum uric acid concentrations in human and it might be one of the possible candidates for the missing link between obesity and hypeuricemia [Bedir et al., 2003].

Uric Acid as a Risk Factor of Cardiovascular Risk in Patients with Metabolic Syndrome

Hyperuricemia, hyperhomocysteinemia, oxidative stress, and inflammation each play an important role in expanding the original concept of MS described by Reaven in the atherosclerotic process. Theses parameters do not stand alone but interacts in a synergistic manner resulting in the progression of accelerated atherosclerosis and endothelial dysfunction [Hayden and Tyagi, 2004].

Although several studies support the role of uric acid as an independent predictor of cardiovascular risk and all-cause mortality [Culleton et al., 1999; Niskanen et al., 2004], uric acid increase has been also considered a component of the metabolic derangement verified in MS in adults [Yoo et al., 2005; Onat et al., 2006] as well as in adolescents and children [Ford et al., 2007]. We have previously reported that MS group of patients presented higher uric acid concentration compared with a healthy control group and that the uric acid had a positive significant correlation with waist circumference, fasting glucose, fasting insulin and HOMA, and a negative significant correlation with HDL-cholesterol [Simão et al., 2008]. The most significant correlation verified, in that work, was between uric acid and insulin resistance. Insulin resistance has been considered the underlying condition that triggers the development of metabolic disturbances in metabolic syndrome. The association between uric acid concentration and insulin resistance is supported by many evidences [Tsouli et al, 2006; Feig et al., 2008]. First, the degree of insulin resistance has been shown to be directly related to uric acid concentration. Second, drugs that improve insulin sensitivity, such as metformin, troglitazone, sibutramine and orlistat can also lower uric acid concentration. Third, after multiple logistic regression analysis, only uric acid concentration and fasting insulin were independent predictors of nonalcoholic fatty liver disease, which is another common characteristic of metabolic syndrome. Fourth, both alcohol and thiazide diuretic agents may contribute to the development of hyperuricemia and insulin resistance, as well as post-menopausal women are more predisposed to both conditions.

Insulin has a physiologic action on renal tubules, causing a reduction in uric acid clearance [Muscelli et al., 1996], what could explain the higher uric acid levels found in MS. Hyperinsulinemia and insulin resistance could lead to both sodium and uric acid renal tubular absorption, by similar physiopathological mechanisms, which in turn could provoke hyperuricemia and hypertension [Facchini et al., 1991]. In addition, insulin may enhance renal urate absorption through stimulation of the urate-anion exchanger urate transporter-1 (URAT1) (Choi et al., 2004). On the other hand, there are several mechanisms by which hypertension can cause hyperuricemia through vascular disease and increased renal vascular resistance: decreased renal blood flow which stimulates urate reabsorption; ischemia leading to lactate release which competes with urate transporter and blocks urate excretion; increased adenosine degradation induced by ischemia and consequent appearance of adenine and xanthine. Xanthine and xanthine oxidase generation lead to increased uric acid production [Tsouli et al., 2006].

Uric Acid and Inflammation in MS

The four players in the MS are hyperinsulinemia, hypertension, hyperlipidemia, and hyperglycemia. Abdominal obesity and insulin resistance are the core features of MS. Inflammation, demonstrated primarily by elevated levels of serum C-reactive protein, is thought to be associated with insulin resistance and MS [Festa et al., 2000; Haffner, 2003; Tamakoshi et al., 2003]. Central obesity is considered to be one of the most important determinants of the low-grade chronic inflammation present in MS [Santos et al., 2005]. Adipose tissue produces proinflammatory cytokines, such as interleukin 6 (IL-6), tumor necrosis factor-α (TNF-α), and complement factors [Trayhurn and Wood, 2004]. However, this tissue also secretes adiponectin, a protein showing anti-inflammatory activity, which inhibits TNF-α production [Yokota et al., 2000], adhesion molecule expression, and nuclear transcriptional factor κB signaling, a pivotal pathway in inflammatory reactions in endothelial cells [Ouchi et al., 1999, Ouchi et al., 2000]. In addition, adiponectin is anti-atherogenic and is an insulin-sensitizing agent [Hotta et al., 2001]. Adipose-derived TNF-α may have negative effects on the expression of adiponectin and vice versa, and these two proteins also have opposite effects on insulin sensitivity [Kern et al., 2001; Maeda et al., 2001]. Given this antagonistic relationship, obesity, and especially visceral obesity, may lead to a decreased secretion of adiponectin through feedback inhibition, thereby suppressing the beneficial effects of adiponectin on insulin sensitivity.

Levels of adiponectin are lower in patients with obesity [Arita et al., 1999], type 2 diabetes mellitus [Hotta et al., 2000], arterial hypertension

[Iwashima et al., 2004] and MS [Xydaki et al., 2004; Santaniemi et al., 2006] Decreases in serum adiponectin levels are associated with different components of MS, and the decreased adiponectin levels appear to be related to increases in the number of MS components in both sexes [Santaniemi et al., 2006].

Uric acid is known to induce the nuclear transcription factor (NF-kappaB) and monocytes chemoattractant protein 1 (MCP-1). Uric acid has also been shown to activate leukocytes and stimulates the production of interleukin 1-β, interleukin 6 (IL-6) and TNF-α by mononuclear cells, and CRP by cultured human vascular cells [Kanellis and Kang, 2005; Waring et al., 2000]. Tamakoshi et al. (2003) have shown a statistically significant positive correlation between CRP and uric acid in a study of 3692 Japanese men. However, in a previous study, our group has not verified any significant association between uric acid levels and inflammatory markers, except for an inverse association with adiponectin [Simão et al., in press], which was also verified in a previous study [Patel et al., 2006]. Lower adiponectin concentration has been considered the link between abdominal fat and insulin resistance in patients predisposed to MS [Santaniemi et al., 2006].

Hyperuricemia in metabolic syndrome is due to underexcretion, and there are many drugs given to hyperuricemia related co-morbidities which have uricosuric properties, such as losartan and anlodipine rather than diuretics for hypertension, fenofibrate for hypertriacylglycerolemia, and metformin to improve insulin sensitivity and for type 2 diabetes mellitus that should be preferentially prescribed in patients with concomitant hyperuricemia [Choi et al., 2004; Tsouli et al., 2006].

Uric Acid as a Component of the Antioxidant Defense System

Uric acid is an important antioxidant, being responsible for 60% of the scavenging activity of the free radicals in human plasma [Cecchini et al., 1990; Ames et al., 1981]. In a previous study, we have verified that patients with the MS showed increased oxidative stress, verified by elevated levels of serum hydroperoxides, whereas total radical-trapping antioxidant parameter (TRAP) did not decrease and TBARS/MDA did not increase probably due to uric acid enhance [Simão et al., 2008]. TRAP may not decrease in diseases in which uric acid concentration may be increased since, in this reaction, the azobis compound generates peroxyl radicals that is scavenged by uric acid with a constant rate of about 10^8 $M^{-1}s^{-1}$ consequently reducing the light emission [Halliwell and Guthridge, 1999]. Therefore, uric acid increase in these conditions, such as metabolic syndrome, for instance, should compensate any reduction in others low molecular weight antioxidants. In the abovementioned study [Simão et al., 2008] the influence of uric acid on oxidative stress and antioxidant mechanisms was reinforced by the following findings: Several components of MS: waist circumference, fasting glucose as well as fasting insulin and insulin resistance (HOMA-IR) showed an inverse significant correlation with TBARS/MDA and a positive significant correlation with uric acid. There was a positive correlation between uric acid levels and total antioxidant capacity, and both parameters correlated positive and concomitantly with waist circumference, fasting insulin and insulin resistance. Nieto et al. (2000) also found higher total antioxidant capacity associated with higher uric acid concentrations among individuals with atherosclerosis and suggested that hyperuricemia may be a compensatory mechanism to counteract oxidative damage related to atherosclerosis in humans. On the other hand, reduced total antioxidant capacity, in obese children with the metabolic syndrome has been observed [Molnár et al., 2004]. However, this assay is based on the reaction between metmyoglobin and hydrogen peroxide, which generates a free radical, therefore quite different from TRAP reaction.

Uric acid may trigger the ROS generation through various mechanisms, for instance, activating the NADPH oxidase system. Sautin et al. has demonstrated this statement in adypocites. ROS increase give raise to $ONOO^-$ by reaction with NO• leading to protein nitrosylation, lipid peroxidation and NO• reduction altering endothelial function. Therefore, uric acid seems to have a double role in oxidative stress measurements.

Relationship between Uric Acid, Oxidative Stress and Endothelial Dysfunction

The upper 1/3 of the normal physiologic–homeostatic range (>4.0mg/dL) and abnormal elevations (>6.5 or 7.0mg/dL in men and >6.0mg/dL in women) in serum uric acid should be considered as one of the multiple injurious stimuli to the arterial vessel wall and capillary, which may contribute to endothelial dysfunction and arterial capillary vessel wall remodelling through oxidative–redox stress [Fang and Alderman, 2000; Niskanen et al., 2004].

Vascular dysfunction and damage have been shown to be associated with impaired endothelial nitric oxide (NO) metabolism and function. Endothelial dysfunction is considered a hallmark in the pathophysiology of MS, and it can be evaluated by several means, including the assessment of NO metabolite (NOx) levels [Williams et al., 2002]. NO is synthesized in endothelial cells by endothelial nitric oxide synthase (eNOS) activity, and it is responsible for vasodilatation and the maintenance of endothelial function; eNOS is expressed constitutively and synthesizes NO in only small amounts under basal conditions. NO production may also be stimulated by an increase in inducible nitric oxide synthase (iNOS) expression, for instance, by oxidative stress or pro-inflammatory cytokines [Natham, 1997]. Therefore, iNOS-derived NO mediates the inflammatory response, and it has been shown to cause vascular dysfunction in a number of experimental models [Gunnet et al., 2003].

A myriad of pathological factors of MS, such as insulin resistance, hyperuricemia, inflammation, hypoadiponectinemia, and oxidative stress could lead to a decrease in NO bioavailability (Williams et al., 2002; Nathan, 1997; Gunnet et al., 2003; Asl et al., 2008). Oxidative redox stress results in impaired endothelium-dependent vasodilation with quenching of endothelial nitric oxide and allows the endothelium to become a net producer of ROS specifically superoxide as the eNOS enzyme uncouples to produce superoxide instead of eNOS (Hayden and Tyagi, 2004). Superoxide also passively increases an inhibitory substrate (asymmetric dimethylarginine) by inhibiting the enzyme, dimethylarginine dymethylaminothydrolase [Forstermann, 2006].

Uric acid can also form free radicals through other reactions, including peroxynitrite whose products are responsible for the amplification of lipid oxidation [Imaram et al., 2010]. In addition, uric acid has been shown to reduce NO bioavailability in various cell types via mechanisms involving redox control [Cecchini et al., 1990] and also activating arginase and depleting NO [Ames et al., 1981]. The uric acid involvement in oxidative and nitroactive stress is very complex because its antioxidant/prooxidant capacity. Probably this balance is concentration and pH dependent. For instance, uric acid was found to scavenge peroxynitrite very effectively in vivo [Kuzkaya et al., 2005] and its conjugate base, urate, inhibits tyrosine nitration. This reaction is pH dependent since peroxynitrite may form peroxynitrous acid (pKa = 6.8) that rapidly undergo hemolysis to yield nitrogen dioxide which is the real responsible for tyrosine nitration and hydroxyl radicals which in turn is strongly lipid peroxidant [Szabo et al., 2007; Augusto et al., 2002]. At the same time, uric acid can form free radicals in various reactions yielding products also responsible for lipid peroxidation, as pointed out before. The uric acid increase together with reactive oxygen species generation may be responsible for the reduced NO levels which in turn leads to endothelial dysfunction. Allopurinol may improve endothelial function, oxidative stress burden, and improve myocardial efficiency by reducing oxygen consumption [George and Stuthers, 2009]. Allopurinol has been shown to improve endothelial function and to decrease MDA in patients with metabolic syndrome [Yiginer et al., 2008]. George et al. [2006] have shown that improvement of endothelial function after allopurinol was due to decreased oxidative stress, and not to urate reduction, and that allopurinol abolished the vitamin C-sensitive component of oxidative stress on vascular endothelial function. The authors suggested that high-dose (600 mg/d) allopurinol would reduce the production of superoxide dismutase and further co-infusion of vitamin C would not find superoxide anions to scavanger. Interestingly, the magnitude of high-dose allopurinol effect on endothelial function was remarkable, and much greater than angiotensin-converting enzyme inhibitors or statins.

Gersch et al. (2008) demonstrated that uric acid reacts directly with NO in a rapid irreversible reaction resulting in the formation of 6-aminouracil and depletion of NO. This reaction occurs preferentially with NO even in the presence of oxidant peroxynitrite and hydrogen peroxide and that the reaction is at least partially blocked by glutathione. This is a potential mechanism by which uric acid may deplete NO and cause endothelial dysfunction, particularly under conditions of oxidative stress in which uric acid is elevated and intracellular gluthatione is depleted.

Determination of thiobarbituric acid reactive substances (TBARS) expressed in μmol malondialdehyde (TBARS/MDA) is probably the most used tool to measure oxidative stress. However, in a system where uric acid increases, as verified in MS, reduced formation of MDA should be expected despite the increased ROOH levels [Simão et al., 2008].This occurs because uric acid reduces organic peroxyl radicals ($ROO^{\bullet}$) into hydroperoxide (ROOH), blockading its degradation to low molecular weight aldehydes, including MDA [Maxwell et al., 1997]. Therefore, in higher uric acid concentration conditions, other oxidative stress measurements, such as analysis of tert-butyl hydroperoxide-initiated chemiluminescence (CL-LOOH) should be used instead [Simão et al., 2008]. Uric acid does not interfere with the ROOH amount previously present in plasma and consequently in the CL levels, because the high tert butyl hydroperoxide concentration (3 mM) against plasmatic uric acid concentration (0.037 mM) in reaction mixture.

This antixodant-prooxidant urate redox shuttle seems to rely heavily on its surrounding environment such as if early or late in the disease process, location of the tissue and substrate, pH, the surrounding oxidant milieu, depletion of other local antioxidant, the supply and duration of oxidant substrate and its oxidant enzyme. In the accelerated atherosclerotic–vulnerable plaque the intima has been shown to be acidic, depleted of local antioxidants with an underlying increase in oxidant stress and ROS and associated with uncoupling of the eNOS enzyme and a decrease in the locally produced naturally occurring antioxidant (Hayden and Tyagi, 2004).

Conclusion and Perspectives

The traditional and innocent role of uric acid increase has been challenged by several reports. As hyperuricemia may favor the development of several metabolic disorders, including metabolic syndrome, all related co-morbidities may be investigated in depth. Although uric acid may have a protective effect due to its antioxidant properties, it is clear that the dominant effect of uric acid in MS is deleterious. It is still unclear which of the following detrimental roles of uric acid is more important: mediating the effects of conventional risk factors in the development of the atherosclerotic disease; mediating the effects of an anti-inflammatory status; or mediating the effects of a pro-inflammatory status. Previous studies which showed an inverse relationship between uric acid levels and adiponectin seem to reinforce the former two hypotheses. Long-term studies to verify the consequences of decreasing uric acid concentration below the present recommendations in asymptomatic patients are warranted.

References

Alper Jr, A.B.; Chen, W.C.; Yau, L.; Srinivasan, S.R.; Berenson, G.S.; Hamm, L.L. Childhood uric acid predicts adult blood pressure (2005). The Bogalusa Heart Study. *Hypertension*, 45, 34-38.

Ames, B.N.; Cathcart, R.; Schwiers, E.; Hochstein, P. (1981) Uric acid provides an antioxidant defense in humans against oxidant-and radical-caused aging and cancer: a hypothesis. *Proc Natl Acad Sci Usa*,. 78, 6858-6862.

Arita, Y.; Kihara, S.; Ouchi, N.; Takahashi, M.; Maeda, K.; Miyagawa, J.; Hotta, K.; Shimomura, I.; Nakamura, T.; Miyaoka, K.; Kuriyama, H.; Nishida, M.; Yamashita, S.; Okubo, K.; Matsubara, K.; Muraguchi, M.; Ohmoto, Y.; Funahashi, T.; Matsuzawa, Y. (1999). Paradoxal decrease of an adipose-specific protein, adiponectin in obesity. *Biochem Biophys Res Commun*, 257, 79-83.

Asl, S.Z.; Ghasemi, A.; Azizi, F. (2008). Serum nitric oxide metabolites in subjects with metabolic syndrome. Clin Biochem, 41, 1342-1347.

Augusto, O.; Bonini, M. G.; Amanso, A. M.; Linares, E.; Santos, C. C. X.; de Menezes, S. L. (2002). Nitrogen dioxide and carbonate radical anion: two emerging radicals in biology. Free Radic Biol. Med, 32, 841–859.

Bedir, A.; Topbas, M.; Tanyeri, F.; Alvur, M.; Arik, N. (2005). Leptin might be a regulator of serum uric acid concentration in humans. Jpn Heart J, 44, 527-536.

Cannon, P.J.; Stason, W.B.; Demartini, F.E.; Sommers, S.C.; Laragh, J.H. (1966). Hypeuricemia in primary and renal hypertension. N Engl J Med, 275, 457-464.

Cecchini, R.; Aruoma, O.I.; Halliwell, B. (1990). The action of hydrogen peroxide on the formation of thiobarbituric acid-reactive material frrom microsomes or from DNA damage by bleomycin or o-phenanthroline. Artefacts in the thiobarbituric acid test. Free Rad Res Commun, 10, :245-258.

Choi, H.K.; Ford, E.S. (2007). Prevalence of the metabolic syndrome in individuals with hyperuricemia. Am J Med, 120, 442-447.

Choi, H.K.; Mount, D.B.; Reginato, A.M. Pathogenesis of gout. (2004). Ann Inter Med, 143, 499-516.

Choi, J.W.; Ford, E.S.; Gao, X.; Choi, H.K. Sugar sweetened soft drinks, diet soft drinks, and serum acid level: The Third National Health and Nutrition Examination Survey. (2008). Arthritis Rheum 59, 109-116.

Cook, S.; Hugli, O.; Egli, M.; Vollenweider, P.; Brucelin, R.; Nicod, P.; Thorens, B.; Scherrer, U. (2003). Clustering of cardiovascular risk factors mimicking the human metabolic syndrome. Swiss Med Wkly, 133, 360-3.

Culleton, B,F,; Larson, M.G.; Kannel, W.B.; Levy, D. (1999). Serum uric acid and risk for cardiovascular disease and death: the Framingham Heart Study. Ann Intern Med, 131, 7-13.

Facchini, F.; Chen, I.; Hollenbeck, C.B.; Reaven, G.M. Relationship between resistance to insulin-mediated glucose uptake, urinary uric acid clearance, and plasma uric concentration. (1991). JAMA, 266, 3008-3011.

Fang, J.; Alderman, M.H. (2000). Serum uric acid and cardiovascular mortality the NHANES I epidemiologic follow-up study, 1971-1992. National Health and Nutrition Examination Survey. JAMA, 283, 2404-2410.

Feig, D.I.; Kang, D.H.; Johnson RJ. (2008). Uric acid and cardiovascular disease. NEJM, 359, 1811-1821.

Festa, A.; D'Agostino, Jr. R.; Howard, G.; Mykkänen, L.; Tracy, R.P.; Haffner, S.M. (2000). Chronic subclinical inflammation as part of the insulin resistance syndrome. The Insulin Resistance Atherosclerosis Study (IRAS). Circulation, 102, 42-47.

Ford, E.S.; Li, C.; Cook, S.; Choi, H.K. (2007). Serum concentrations of uric acid and the metabolic syndrome among US children and adolescents. Circulation, 115, 2526-2532.

Forstemann, U. (2006). Janus-faced role of endothelial NO synthase in vascular disease: Uncoupling of oxygen reduction from NO synthesis and its pharmacological reversal. Biol Chem, 387, 1521-1533.

Gagliardi, A.C.M.; Minamc, M.H.; Santos, R.D. (2009). Uric acid: a marker of increased cardiovascular risk. Atherosclerosis, 202, 11-17.

George, J.; Carr, E.; Davies, J.; Belch, J.J.F.; Stuthers, A. (2006). High-dose allopurinol improves endothelial function by profoundly reducing vascular oxidative stress and not by lowering uric acid. Circulation, 114, 2508-2516.

George, J.; Stuthers, A.D. (2009). Role of urate, xanthine oxidase and the effects of allopurinol in vascular oxidative stress. Vasc Health Risk Manag, 5, 265-272.

Gercsh, C.; Palii, S.P.; Kim, K.M.; Angerhofer, A.; Johnson, R.J.; Henderson, G.N. (2008). Inactivation of nitric oxide by uric acid. Nucleosides Nucleotides Nucleic Acids, 27, 967-978.

Gunnett, C.A.; Heistad, D.D.; Faraci, F.M. (2003). Gene target mice reveal a critical role for inducible nitric oxide synthase in vascular dysfunction during diabetes. Stroke, 34, 2970-2974.

Haffner, S.M. (2003). Insulin resistance, inflammation and the prediabetic state. Am J Cardiol 92, 18-26J.

Halliwell, B.; Gutteridge, J.M.C. Antioxidant protection by compounds synthesized in vivo, third ed., Oxford University Press, New York., page 19, 197, 1999.

Hayden, M.R.; Tyagi, S.C. (2004). Uric acid: A new look at an old risk marker for cardiovascular disease, metabolic syndrome, and the diabetes mellitus: The urate redox shuttle. Nutrition and Metabolism, 1, 1-10- .

Ho, W-J.; Tsai, W-P.; Yu, K-H.; Tsay, P-K.; Wang, C-L.; Hsu, T-S.; Kuo, C-T. (2010). Association between endothelial function and hyperuricemia. Rheumatology, 49, 1929-1934.

Hotta, K.; Funahashi, T.; Arita, Y.; Takahashi, M.; Matsuda, M.; Okamoto, Y.; Iwahashi, H.; Kuriyama, H.; Ouchi, N.; Maeda, K.; Nishida, M.; Kihara, S.; Sakai, N.; Nakajima, T.; Hasegawa, K.; Muraguchi, M.; Ohamoto, Y.; Nakamura, T.; Yamashita, S.; Hanafusa, T.; Matsuzawa, Y. (2000). Plasma concentrations of a novel, adipose-specific protein, adiponectin, in type 2 diabetic patients. Artherioscler Thromb Vasc Biol, 20, 1595-1599.

Hotta, K.; Funahashi, T.; Bodkin, N.L.; Ortmeyer, H.K.; Arita, Y.; Hansen, B.C.; Matsuzawa, Y. (2001). Circulating concentrations of the adipocyte protein adiponectin are decreased in parallel with reduced insulin sensitivity during the progress to type 2 diabetes in rhesus monkeys. Diabetes, 50, 1126-1133.

Hovind, P.; Rossing, P.; Tarnow, L.; Johnson, R.J.; Parving, H.H. (2009). Serum acid uric as a predictor for development of diabetic nephropathy in type 1 diabetes. Diabetes, 58, 1668-1671.

Imaram, W.; Gersch, C.; Kim, K.M.; Johnson, R.J.; Henderson, G.N.; Angerhofer, A. (2010). Radicals in the reaction between peroxynitrite and uric acid identified by electron spin resonance spectroscopy and liquid chromatography mass spectrometry. Free Radic Biol Med, 49, 275-281.

Iwashima, Y.; Katsuya, T.; Ishikawa, K.; Ouchi, N.; Ohishi, M.; Sugimoto, K.; Fu, Y.; Motone, M.; Yamamoto, K.; Matsuo, A.; Ohashi, K.; Kihara, S.; Funahashi, T.; Rakugi, H.; Matsuzawa, Y.; Ogihara, T. (2004). Hypoadiponectinemia is an independent risk factor for hypertension. Hypertension, 43, 1318-1323.

Johnson, R.J.; Feig, D.I.; Herrera-Acosta, J.; Kang, D-H. (2005a). Resurrection of uric acid as a causal risk factor in essential hypertension. Hypertension, 45, 18-20.

Johnson, R.J.; Herrera-Acosta, J.; Screiner, GF.; Rodriguez-Iturbe, B. (2002a). Subtle acquired renal injury as a mechanism of salt sensitive hypertension. N Engl J Med, 346, 913-923.

Johnson, R.J.; Rodriguez-Iturbe, B.; Kang, D-H.; Feig, D.I.; Herrera-Acosta, J. (2005b). A unifying pathway for essential hypertension. Am J Hypertens, 18, 431-440.

Kanellis, J.; Kang, D.H. (2005). Uric acid as a mediator of endothelial dysfunction, inflammation, and vascular disease. Sem Nephrol, 25, 39-43.

Kern, P.A.; Ranganathan, S.; Li, C.; Wood, L.; Ranganathan, G. (2001). Adipose tissue tumor necrosis factor and IL-6 expression in human obesity and insulin resistance. Am J Physiol Endocrinol Metab, 280, E745-751.

Khosla, U.M.; Zharikov, S.; Finch, J.L.; Nakagawa, T.; Roncal, C.; Mu, W.; Krotova, K.; Block, E.R.; Prabhakar, S.; Johnson, RJ. (2005). Hyperuricemia induces endothelial dysfunction. Kidney Intern, 67, 1739-1742.

Koprovski, H.; Spitsin, S.V.; Hooper, D.C. Prospects for the treatment of multiple sclerosis by raising serum levels of uric acid, a scavenger of peroxynitrite. [2001]. Ann Neurol, 49:139.

Kuzkaya, N.;Weissmann, N.; Harrison, D. G.; Dikalov, S. (2005). Interactions of peroxynitrite with uric acid n the presence of ascorbate and thiols: implications for uncoupling endothelial nitric oxide synthase. Biochem Pharmacol, 70, 343–354.

Lin, K.C.; Tsao, H.M.; Chen, C.H.; Chou, P. (2004). Hypertension was the major risk factor leading to development of cardiovascular diseases among men with hyperuricemia. J Rheumatol, 31,1152-1158.

Maeda,, N.; Takahashi, M.; Funahashi, Y.; Kihara, S.; Nishizawa, H.; Kishida, K.; Nagaretani, H.; Matsuda, M.; Komuro, R.; Ouchi, N.; Kuriyama, H.; Hotta, K.; Nakamura, T.; Shimomura, I.; Matsuzawa, Y. (2001). PPAR-γ ligands increase expression and plasma concentration of adiponectin, an adipose-driven protein. Diabetes, 50, 2094-2099.

Maxwell, S.R.; Thomason, H.; Sandler, D.; LeGuen, C.; Baxter, M.A.; Thorpe, G.H.; Jones, A.F.; Barnett, A.H. (1997). Antioxidant status in patients with uncomplicated insulin-dependent and non-insulin-dependent diabetes mellitus. Eur J Clin Invest, 27, 484-490.

Mazzali, M.; Hughes, J.; Kim, Y.G.; Jefferson, J. A.; Kamg, D-H.; Gordon, K.L.; Lan, H.Y.; Kivlighn, S.; Johnson, R.J. (2001). Elevated uric acid increases blood pressure in the rat by a novel crystal-independent mechanism. Hypertension, 38, 1101-1106.

Mené, P.; Punzo, G. (2008). Uric acid: bystander or culprit in hypertension and progressive renal disease? J Hypertens, 26, 2085-2092.

Mercuro, G.; Vitale, C.; Cerquetani, E.; Zancu, S.; Deidda, M.; Fine, M.; Rosano, G.M.C. (2004). Effect of hyperuricemia upon endothelial function in patients at increased cardiovascular risk. Am J Cadiol, 94, 932-935.

Molnár, D.; Decsil, T.; Koletzko, B. (2004). Reduced antioxidant status in obese children with multimetabolic syndrome. Intern J Obesity, 28, 1197-1202.

Muscelli, E.; Natali, A.; Bianchi, S.; Bigazzi, R.; Galvan, A.Q.; Sironi, A.M.; Franscerra, S.; Ciociaro, D.; Ferrannini, E. (1996) Effect of insulin on renal sodium and uric acid handling in essential hypertension. Am J Hypertens, 9, 746-752.

Nakagawa, T.; Hu, H.; Zharikov, S.; Tutle, K.R.; Short, R.A.; Glushakova, O.; Ouyang, X.; Feig, D.I.; Block, E.R.; Herrera-Acosta, J.; Patel, J.M.; Johnson, R.J. (2006). A causal role for uric acid in fructose-induced metabolic syndrome. Am J Physiol Renal Physiol, 290, F625-631.

Nathan C. (1997). Inducible nitric oxide synthase: what difference does it make? J Clin Invest, 100, 2417-2423.

Nieto, F.J.; Iribarren, C.; Gross, M.D.; Comstock., G.W.; Cutler, R.G. (2000). Uric acid and serum antioxidant capacity: a reaction to atherosclerosis? Atherosclerosis, 148, 131-139.

Niskanen, L.K.; Laaksonen, D.E.; Nyyssonen, K.; Alfthan, G.; Lakka, H.M.; Lakka, T.A.,; Salonen, J.T. (2004). Uric acid level as a risk for cardiovascular and all-mortality in middle-age men: a prospective cohort study. Arch Intern Med, 164, 1546-1551.

Onat, H.; Uyarel, H.; Hergenç, G.; Karabulut, A.; Albayrak, S.; Sari, I.; Yazici, M.; Keles, I. (2006). Serum acid is a determinant of metabolic syndrome in a population-based study. Am J Hypertens 19, 1055-1062.

Ouchi, N.; Kihara, S.; Arita, Y.; Okamoto, Y.; Maeda, K.; Kuriyama, H.; Hotta, K.; Nishida, M.; Takahashi, M.,; Nakamura, T.; Yamashita, S.; Funahashi, T.; Matsuzawa, Y. (1999). Novel modulator for endothelial adhesión molecules: Adipocyte-derived plasma protein adiponectin. Circulation, 100, 2473-2476.

Ouchi, N.; Kihara, S.; Arita, Y.; Okamoto, Y.; Maeda, K.; Kuriyama, H.; Hotta, K.; Nishida, M.; Takahashi, M.; Muraguchi, M.; Ohmoto, Y.; Nakamura, T.; Yamashita, S.; Funahashi, T.; Matsuzawa, Y. (2000). Adiponectin, an adipocyte-derived plasma protein, inhibits endothelial NF-kappaB signaling through a cAMP-dependent pathway. Circulation, 102, 1296-1301.

Patel, D.A.; Srinivasan, S.R.; Xu, J.H..; Chen, W.; Berenson, G.S. (2006). Adiponectin and its correlates of cardiovascular risk in young adults: the Bogalusa Heart Study. Metab Clin Exp, 55, 1551-7.

Sánchez-Lozada, L.G.; Nakagawa, T.; Kang, D-H; Feig, D.I.; Franco, M.; Johson, R.J.; Herrera-Acosta, J. (2006). Hormonal and cytokine effects of uric acid. Curr Opin Nephrol Hypertens, 15, 30-33.

Sanchéz-Lozada, L.G.; Tapia, E.; Bautista-Garcia, P.; Soto, V.; Ávila-Casado, C.; Veja-Campos, I.P.; Nakagawa, T.; Zhao, L.; Franco, M.; Johnson, R.J.

(2008). Effects of febuxostat on metabolic and renal alterations in rats with fructose-induced metabolic syndrome. Am J Physiol Renal Physiol, 294, F710-718.

Santaniemi, M.; Kesäniemi, Y.A.; Ukkola, O. (2006). Low plasma adiponectin concentration is an indicator of the metabolic syndrome. Eur J Endocr, 155, 745-750.

Santos, A.C.; Lopes, C.; Guimarães, J.T.; Barros, H. (2005). Central obesity as a major determinant of increased high-sensitivity C-reactive protein in metabolic syndrome. Intern J Obes, 29, 1452-1456.

Sautin, Y.Y.; Nakagawa, T.; Zharikov, S.; Johnson, R.J. (2007) Adverse effects of the classic antioxidant uric acid in adipocytes: NADPH oxidase-mediated oxidative/nitrosative stress Am J Physiol Cell Physiol, 293, C584-596.

Simão, A.N.C.; Dichi, J.B.; Barbosa, D.S.; Cecchini, R.; Dichi, I. (2008). Influence of uric acid and γ-glutamyltransferase on total antioxidant capacity and oxidative stress in patients with metabolic syndrome. Nutrition, 24, 675-681.

Simão, A.N.C.; Lozovoy, M.A.B.; Simão, T.N.C.; Morimoto, H.K.; Dichi, I. (in press). Adiponectinemia is associated with uricemia but not with proinflammatory status in women with metabolic syndrome. J Nutr Metab.

Sundström, J.; Sullivan, L.; D`Agostino, R.B.; Levy, D.; Kannel, W.B.; Vasan, R.S. (2005). Relations of serum uric acid to longitudinal blood pressure tracking and hypertension incidence. Hypertension, 45, 28-33.

Szabo, C.; Ischiropoulos, H.; Radi, R. (2007). Peroxynitrite: biochemistry, pathophysiology and development of therapeutics. Nat Rev Drug Discovery 6, 662–680.

Tamakoshi, K.; Yatsuya, H.; Kondo, T.; Hori, Y.; Ishikawa, M.; Zhang, H.; Murata, C.; Otsuka, R.; Zhu, S.; Toyoshima, H. (2003). The metabolic syndrome is associated with elevated circulating C-reactive protein in healthy reference range, a systemic low-grade inflammatory state. Int J Obes Relat Metab Disord, 27, 443– 449.

Trayhurn, P.; Wood, I.S. (2004). Adipokines: inflammation and the pleiotropic role of the white adipose tissue. Br J Nutr, 92, 347-355.

Tsouli, S.G.; Liberopoulos, E.N.; Mikhailidis, D.P.; Athyros, V.G.; Elisaf, M.S. (2006). Elevated uric acid levels in metabolic syndrome: an active component or an innocent bystander? Metab Clin Exp 55, 1293-1301.

Waring, W.S.; Webb, D.J.; Maxwell, S.R.J. (2000). Uric acid as a risk factor for cardiovascular disease. Q J Med, 93, 707-713.

Watanabe, S.; Kang, D-H.; Feng, L.; Nakagawa, T.; Kannelis, L.; Lan, H.; Mazzali, M.; Johnson, R.J. (2002b). Uric acid, hominoid evolution, and the pathogenesis salt-sensitivity. Hypertension, 40, 355-360.

Williams, I.L.; Wheatcroft, S.B.; Shah, A.M.; Kearney, M.T. (2002). Obesity, atherosclerosis and the vascular endothelium: mechanism of reduced nitric oxide bioavailability in obese human. Int J Obes, 26, 754-764.

Xydaki AM, Case CC, Jones PH, Hoogeveen RC, Liu M, O'Brian SE.; Nelson, K.W.; Ballantyne, C.M. (2004). Adiponectin, inflammation, and the expression of the metabolic syndrome in obese individuals: the impact of rapid weight loss through caloric restriction. J Clin Endocrinol Metab, 89, 2697-2703.

Yiginer, O.; Ozcelik, F.; Inanc, T.; Aparci, M.; Ozmen, N.; Cingozbay, B.Y.; Kardesoglu, E.; Suleymanoglu, S.; Sener, G.; Cebeci, B. (2008). Allopurinol improves endothelial function and reduces oxidant-inflammatory enzyme of myeloperoxidase in metabolic syndrome. Clin Res Cardiol, 97, 334-340.

Yokota, T.; Oritani, K.; Takahashi, I.; Ishikawa, J.; Matsuyama, A.; Ochi, N.; Kihara, S.; Funashi, T.; Tenner, A.J.; Tomiyama, Y.; Matsuzawa, Y. (2000). Adiponectin, a new member of the family of soluble defense collagens, negatively regulates the growth of mielomonocytic progenitors and the functions of the macrophages. Blood, 96, 1723-1732.

Yoo, T.W.; Sung, K.C.; Shin, H.S.; Kim, B.J.; Kim, B.S.; Kang, J.H.; Lee, M.H.; Park, J.R.; Kim, H. Rhee, E.J.; LEE, w.y.; Kim, S.W.; Ryu, S.H.; Keum, D.G. (2005). Relationship between serum uric acid concentration and insulin resistance and metabolic syndrome. Cir J, 69, 928-933.

Zavaroni, I.; Mazza, S.; Fantuzzi, M.; Dall'Aglio, E.; Bonora, E.; Delsignore, R.; Passeri, M.; Reaven, G.M. (1993). Changes in insulin and lipid metabolism in males with asymptomatic hypeuricaemia. J Intern Med, 234, 25-30.

In: Uric Acid
Editors: S. Castillo and E. Maldonado
ISBN 978-1-62100-762-3

Chapter IV

The Role of Serum Uric Acid in Hypertension and Renal Failure: Is a Marker or the Cause?

Chung-Sheng Lin [*]
Department of Internal Medicine, Chung Shan Medical University Hospital and School of Medicine, Chung Shan Medical University, Taichung, Taiwan

Abstract

Clinical evidence suggests that hyperuricemia is an important, independent risk factor for cardiovascular renal disease and hypertension. A post-hoc analysis of hypertension clinical trials has also shown that patients with lower serum uric acid levels have a better outcome after reducing their blood pressure with anti-hypertensive drugs. Evidence from a cross-sectional study found that serum uric acid levels were significantly linear, corresponding to serum creatinine levels and

[*] Address for correspondence: Chung-Sheng Lin M.D., Department of Internal Medicine, Chung Shan Medical University Hospital, 110, Section 1, Chien Kuo North Road, Taichung, Taiwan 402, Phone 886-4-24739595 #34711, Fax: 886-4-24739220, E-mail: lcs@csmu.edu.tw

suggesting that serum uric acid may play an intermediate role in reflecting renal function; this may be regarded as representing serum creatinine in renal failure progression in hypertensive subjects. Nevertheless, a recent animal study had demonstrated that uric acid may produce hypertension and renal failure by inducing vascular endothelial damage and produce vascular dysfunction, thus activating the renin angiotensin system.

However, controversy exists, due to the lack of clinical evidence, to explore the causal effect between uric acid and hypertension development.

Therefore, it is still not yet known whether serum uric acid is the cause or the marker of the hypertension and renal failure. Clinical trials are needed to determine if a uric acid lowering therapy would be effective in preventing renal failure and hypertension.

Introduction

Over the past decade, a substantial body of clinical evidence has accumulated suggesting that hyperuricemia is an important, independent risk factor for cardiovascular and renal disease; not only in patients with hypertension [1-8], heart failure [9], or diabetes [10], but also in the general population [11-12]. Patients with hypertension and hyperuricemia have a significant risk of target organ damage. Particularly, women have a 75% higher risk of having cardiac hypertrophy, and a 2-times greater risk of having carotid abnormalities [13]. Despite blood pressure control, serum uric acid levels increased during treatment and were significantly and directly associated with cardiovascular events, independent of diuretic use and other cardiovascular risk factors [14].

Meta-analyses suggested that hyperuricemia may modestly increase the risks of both stroke incidence [relative risk (RR) 1.41] and mortality (RR 1.36) [15].

The Framingham Study [16] demonstrated that serum uric acid was an independent predictor of hypertension incidence and longitudinal blood pressure progression. Nevertheless, the strong association of serum uric acid and cardiovascular diseases does not imply a causal relationship between them.

Clinical observation results raise the questions of the possibility that uric acid lowering therapies may have some utility in preventing cardiovascular renal disease, and whether serum uric acid is a maker or the cause in the cardiovascular renal disease.

This review will primarily focus on this issue and discuss the interrelationship of serum uric acid to hypertension and cardiovascular renal disease.

Potential Impact of Uric Acid on Hypertension - Epidemiology

Hyperuricemia is commonly observed in patients with hypertension, with up to 25% of untreated hypertensives possessing increased levels of serum uric acid [5]. Hypertension subjects have a higher prevalence of hyperuricemia: 1.5-fold in men and 1.7-fold in women than that of the general population [17]. In Taiwanese hypertensive men and women, the effect of age on mean serum uric acid levels is changed minimally, except for younger age hypertensives (20-40 years) who have much higher serum uric acid levels than older populations [17]. Ethnic difference is noted with a higher median serum uric acid level in black people than in white [18]; Taiwanese aborigines have a higher prevalence rate of hyperuricemia than the non-aborigine [19]. The serum uric acid level, among women, has a significantly higher predictive value than does with the men, as related to all-causes mortality and ischemic heart disease [18]. Vast of epidemiologic studies suggest that higher serum uric acid increase the risk in predicting hypertension development 1.2-fold to 3-fold (Table 1).

Study results from the Framingham Study [20] showed that the serum uric acid level was an independent predictor of hypertension incidence and longitudinal blood pressure progression. The incidence rate of hypertension increased progressively from 9.8% for the lowest quartile to 15.6% for the highest quartile of serum uric acid; blood pressure progression rates increased from 32.8% (lowest quartile) to 39.6% (top quartile). The Multiple Risk Factor Intervention Trial (MRFIT) [21] also showed that normotensive men, with baseline hyperuricemia, had an 80% excess risk for incident hypertension [hazard ratio (HR) 1.81, 95% confident interval (CI) 1.59 to 2.07], compared to those who did not. Each unit increase in serum uric acid was associated with a 9% increase in the risk for incident hypertension (HR 1.09, 95% CI 1.02 to 1.17).

Table 1. Hyperuricemia predicts hypertension development.

Author	Year Published	Study Size	Follow-Up (years)	Increased Risk
Israel ischemic heart disease study Kahn et al.. [50]	1972	10,000 men	5	2-fold
Kaiser Permanente Selby et al. [20]	1990	2,062 adults	6	3-fold
Utah Hunt et al. [51].	1991	1,482 adults	7	2-fold
Olivetti Heart Jossa et al. [52]	1994	619 men	12	1.2-fold
Osaka Health Survey Taniguchi et al. [53]	2001	6,356 men	10	2-fold
Osaka Factory Masuo et al. [54]	2003	433 men	5	+27 mmHg in systolic BP per each 1-mg/dl change in uric acid
Osaka Health Survey Nakanishi et al. [55]	2003	2,310 men	6	1.6-fold
Okinawa Nagahama et al. [71]	2004	4,489 adults	23	1.5-fold in men 1.9-fold in women
Framingham Heart Sundström et al. [16]	2005	3,329 adults	4	1.17-fold
Bogalusa Heart Alper Jr. et al. [56]	2005	679children	11	Predicts diastolic hypertension
The Normative Aging Study Perlstein et al. [57]	2006	2,062 men	21.5	1.10-fold
ARIC Mellen et al. [58]	2006	9,104 adults	9	1.1-folds
Beaver Dan Health Survey Shankar et al. [59]	2006	25,200 adults	10	1.65-folds
Health Professionals' Follow-up Forman et al. [60]	2007	750 men	8	1.02-fold
MRFIT Krishnan et al. [61]	2007	3,073 men	6	1.1-fold
Nurses' Health Study Forman et al. [62]	2009	1,496 women	8	1.25-fold
The Qingdao Port Health and Nutrition Examination Survey in China Zhang et al. [63]	2009	7,220	4	men 1.55-fold women 1.85-fold

Inter-Relationship of Uric Acid and Risk of Cardiovascular Diseases in Hypertension Subjects

Several epidemiological studies have clearly demonstrated a link, in patients with hypertension, between serum uric acid and cardiovascular diseases. For example, the Worksite Treatment Program [5] demonstrated that a 1mg/dL increase in serum uric acid was associated with a 32% increase in cardiovascular events, a value comparable to the cardiovascular effects of a 46 mg/dL change in total cholesterol or a 10 mmHg change in systolic blood pressure. Similarly, published analyses of the Progetto Ipertensione Umbria Monitoraggio Ambulatoriale (PIUMA) study [3], a 12-year study of 1,720 previously untreated hypertensive patients, revealed that serum uric acid was a powerful predictor of cardiovascular disease and all-cause mortality. After adjusting for a wide variety of confounding variables, patients with uric acid levels in the highest quartile had a increased risk of cardiovascular events (RR 1.73, 95% CI 1.01 to 3.00), fatal cardiovascular events (RR 1.96, 95% CI 1.02 to3.79), and all-cause mortality (RR 1.63, 95% CI 1.02 to 2.57) compared with patients whose uric acid levels were in the second quartile. An 11.9 years follow-up study of 1,423 Finnish middle-age men, initially without cardiovascular disease, had shown a 2.5-fold increase of cardiovascular death and 1.7-fold increase of all-cause death of the upper tertian serum uric acid levels, compare to the lowest tertian [22]. In clinical trials, the serum uric acid-lowering effect of losartan was claimed to contribute to the Losartan Intervention For Endpoint reduction in hypertension (LIFE) [2], estimated that approximately 29% (p=0.004) of the benefit of a losartan-based versus atenolol-based therapy on the composite endpoint of death, myocardial infarction, or stroke may be the result of the differences in achieved serum uric acid levels. Nevertheless, no matter how strong the indication of a relationship between serum uric acid and hypertension or cardiovascular events, we cannot interpret it as one of cause and effect. Therefore, whether serum uric acid is the marker or the casual of hypertension remains to be fully delineated. However, it is possible that hypertension may indirectly elevate serum uric acid by increasing levels of serum lactate [23]. According to this hypothesis, hypertension would produce renal microvascular disease and local tissue hypoxia. This, in turn, would increase levels of serum lactate, which would tend to decrease the tubular secretion of uric acid, thereby producing elevated serum uric acid levels. The increase of serum uric acid in hypertension may also be due to a decrease in the renal blood flow that accompanies the hypertension state, a decrease that may stimulate uric acid reabsorption [24]. Nevertheless, recent novel animal model studies have reported that hyperuricemia induces systemic hypertension and renal injury via crystal-independent mechanis, involving renal vasoconstriction mediated by endothelial dysfunction and activation of the renin-angiotensin system [25]. This proposal mechanism in the animal model study, however, requires a lowering serum acid clinical trial to affirm it. A small scale clinical trial using allopurinol therapy, a serum uric acid lowering agent by inhibiting the enzyme xanthine oxidase, significantly decreases serum uric acid levels in hyper-uricemic patients with mild to moderate chronic kidney disease; but there were no significant differences in systolic or diastolic blood pressure at the end of the study when comparing the two groups [26]. A study of 30 adolescents with hyperuricemia and hypertension, treated with allopurinol, was associated with a significant reduction in both office and ambulatory blood pressure, and the reduction was similar in magnitude to that achieved by most antihypertensive agents [27]. Thus, conflicts of clinical study results are observed. Clinical evidences have yet to show that lowering serum uric acid reduces blood pressure or cardiovascular events.

Renal Handling of Uric Acid

Uric acid is produced in the liver from the degradation of dietary and endogenously synthesized purine compounds. The major modes of uric acid handling have been characterized, including: filtration, reabsorption, secretion, and post-secretory reabsorption. Although uric acid is freely filtered, it is also extensively reabsorbed (98-100%) in the early proximal tubule. This is followed by a tubular secretion in the S2 segment of the proximal tubule, and this secretory process is responsible for most excreted uric acid; the fractional uric acid excretion averaging between 7 and 12% in humans (Figure 1). This indicates that urinary uric acid is predominantly a derivative of tubular secretion [28]. Hyperuricemia usually is secondary to decreased excretion, or increased production. In patients with kidney dysfunction, there is a decreased uric acid urinary excretion, possibly causing hyperuricemia. Uric acid may also elevate indirectly by hypertension induced local tissue hypoxia, increasing levels of serum lactate and decreasing tubular excretion [23].

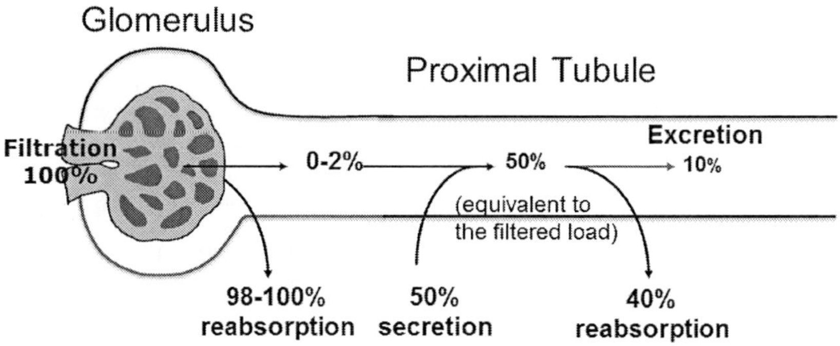

Figure1. Renal handling of uric acid.

Potential Impact of Uric Acid on Chronic Kidney Disease- Epidemiology

A number of recent epidemiology studies have evaluated the association between serum uric acid and prevalent or progressive renal disease, suggesting the independent role of uric acid in renal disease (Table 2). The US Renal Data System (USRDS) database, evaluated 177, 570 patients, followed over 25 years. Patients in the highest quartile of serum uric acid had a hazard ratio of 2.14 for chronic kidney disease [29]. The Vienna Health Screening project evaluated 21,457 subjects and found that an increase in serum uric acid by 2mg/dL conferred and increased the odds ratio of 1.69 of declining renal function [30]. The Okinawa Health Study of 6,403 aged subjects in which the serum uric acid >8mg/dL was associated with a 3-fold increase of end-stage renal disease in men, and more than 10-fold in women [71]. See and colleagues analyzed 28,745 younger subjects, ages 20-49, who underwent routine health screenings in Taiwan. As in the cardiovascular health study, the independent association to incident chronic kidney disease was weak, but uric acid was closely associated with metabolic syndrome and obesity [32]. Lin and colleagues reported that in 2,145 hypertension subjects, serum creatinine had significantly independently predicted serum uric acid elevation (OR 1.759, 95% CI 1.423 to 2.170). Furthermore, in the non-diuretic user group, the highest serum uric acid quartile (>8 mg/dL) entailed >4 times greater risk for serum creatinine elevation than the lowest. In the diuretic user group, a >2 times greater risk was noted [17].

Table 2. Epidemiology of serum uric acid and chronic kidney disease

Author	Year Published	Study Size	Follow-up (years)	Increased Risk
Ben-Dov IZ et al. [35]	2011	2,249	24-28	Hyperuricemia (male>6.5mg/d, female>5.3 mg/dL) increase mortality 1.36-fold, 2.14-fold chronic renal failure and 2.87-fold acute renal failure
Lin CS et al. [33]	2009	2,145 hypertension patients	-	Non diuretic user: uric acid >8 mg/dL increase >4 times greater risk of creatinine elevation Diuretic user: a 2 times greater risk was noted.
Daoussis D et al. [64]	2009	350 rheumatoid arthritis patients		Uric acid is a strong correlate of renal dysfunction in rheumatoid arthritis patients
Hovind P et al. [65]	2009	223 Type 1 DM patients	18.1	uric acid was associated with subsequent development of persistent macroalbuminuria 2.37-fold per 100 mol/l increase in uric acid level
Hsu CY et al. [29]	2009	177,570	25	2.14-fold
Obermaryr RP et al. [30] Vienna Health Screening Project	2008	21,457 adults	-	1.74-fold in men , 3.12-fold in women
Weiner DE et al. [66] , ARIC	2008	13,338		Each 1 mg/dL increase in uric acid increase risk by 7-11%
Iseki K et al. [31] Okinawa	2001	6403		Uric acid >8mg/dl increase CKD risk 3-fold in men and 10-fold in women
Borges RL et al. [49]	2009	385 women		2.63-fold
Chen N et al. [67] China	2009	2,596		Linear correlation between uric acid and degree of CKD
Chen YC et al. [68] Taiwan	2009	5,722		Uric acid associated with prevalent CKD in elderly
Park JT et al. [69]	2009	134		Uric acid >7 mg/dL correlates with more rapid decline in residual renal function in peritoneal dialysis patients
Sturm G et al. [70], MMKD syudy	2008	227		Uric acid predicted progression of CKD only in unadjusted sample
Chonchol, M et al. [34] Cardiovascular Health Study	2007	5,808		Uric acid strongly associated with prevalent but weakly with incident CKD
See LC et al. [32]	2009	28,745		Uric acid >7.7 mg/dL in men and >6.6 mg/dL in women only weakly associated with prevalent renal impairment (-)
Madero M et al. [37]	2009	840		Patients with CKD 3-4 and uric acid correlates with death but not to ESRD

CKD: chronic kidney disease; ESRD: end stage renal disease.

The Role of Uric Acid in Chronic Kidney Disease Progression

The most difficult aspect of assessing uric acid's role in the development or progression of chronic kidney disease is associated with the number of confounders to any study. Because uric acid is predominantly cleared by the kidneys, the decline in renal plasma flow and uric acid excretion will almost universally be associated with increased serum uric acid. The recent clinical study of Lin and colleagues [33] suggested that serum uric acid may play an intermediate role in reflecting renal functioning which may be regarded as representing serum creatinine in renal failure progression. According to their studied 2,145 hypertensive subjects, it was revealed that after an adjusted multivariate, serum creatinine was a strong independent predictor for serum uric acid, and the 4 quartiles of serum uric acid levels were significantly corresponding to serum creatinine concentration in each gender and their subgroups of diuretic users and nonusers (Figure 2). This result is consistent with the study of Chonchol et al. [34], an evaluation of 5,808 adults in the Cardiovascular Health Study, and finding that the estimated glomerular filtration rate was linearly associated with increasing quintiles of uric acid but not with incident chronic kidney disease. There was a weak but statistically significant correlation between uric acid and the progression of chronic kidney disease. In Jerusalem, Ben-Dov [35] studied 2,249 normal baseline kidney function subjects, followed for 24–28 years, and showed that serum uric acid predicted renal failure incidence and all-cause mortality, independently of demographic and glomerular filtration rate. In Japan, Iseki [36] studied community-based screening cohorts, showing that screenees with hyper-uricemia were associated with a greater incidence of end-stage renal disease, and that hyperuricemia was an independent predictor of end-stage renal disease in women. However, in a study of 840 adults with chronic kidney disease, uric acid was closely correlated with all-cause mortality, but not independently with progression to chronic kidney disease [37]. There is very little data which evaluates the efficacy of uric acid reduction on the progression of chronic kidney disease. Kanbay and colleagues [38] treated 48 hyperuricemic and 21 normal uric acid patients, all of whom had normal renal functioning. Fifty-nine patients completed the 3 month study in which they were treated, once daily, with 300mg of allopurinol. With a mean fall in serum uric acid from 8 to 5.5mg/dL, the calculated glomerular filtration rate increased from 79 to 92 ml/min in the hyperuricemic patients, with no change in the control patients. There was no long term follow-up study of the hypouricemic agent on progressive renal disease. Siu and colleagues [39] performed a randomized study of 54 patients with chronic kidney disease, and serum uric acid >7.6 mg/dL to allopurinol or control groups. After 12 months of therapy, 16% of the allopurinol group met the combined endpoint of an increase in serum creatinine of >40%, or initiation of dialysis or death, compared to 46% of the control group. There were no statistically significant differences in blood pressure between the groups. There was not a statistically significant difference in serum creatinine as a continuous variable, but the study was not powered to detect this endpoint. Although there are mixed literatures on the role of allopurinol lowering uric acid levels on the progression of kidney disease, both positive and negative results reported. Care should be taken whether the mechanism of the slowing kidney progression is attributing to lowering the serum uric acid or due to xanthine oxides inhibition, or both. Xanthine oxidase plays an important role in producing oxidative stress. Allopurinol, a xanthine oxidase inhibitor, has been shown to improve endothelial dysfunction, reduce the oxidative stress burden and improve myocardial efficiency by reducing oxygen consumption in smaller mechanistic studies [40]. A recent study [41] of the clinical benefits of oxypurinol, a xanthine oxidase inhibitor, in heart failure patients has shown that oxypurinol did not produce clinical improvements in unselected patients with moderate-to-severe heart failure. However, a post-hoc analysis suggests that benefits occur in patients with elevated serum uric acid in a manner correlating with the degree of serum uric acid reduction. Authors suggested that serum uric acid may serve as a valuable biomarker to target xanthine oxidase inhibition in heart failure.

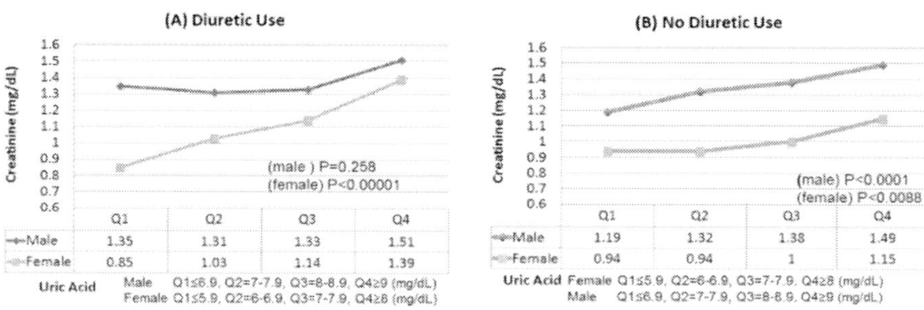

Figure 2. Correlation of serum uric acid and serum creatinine concentrations in hypertension treated patients by gender and diuretic use (reproduce form table 3 of reference 33, P value represent trend test, Q=quartile).

Potential Impact of Diuretic Use on Serum Uric Acid and Renal Function

Diuretics are highly recommended for hypertensive treatment by guidelines, in spite of which may elevate serum uric acid concentration. A study showed that in 438 hypertensive patients receiving diuretics, hyper-uricemia occurred in 44% of those receiving thiazides, 56% of those receiving loop diuretics, and 57% of those receiving aldosterone receptor blockers [33]. Much concern is regarding whether diuretics induce renal function impairment. Previous hypotheses suggested that diuretic use may deplete the renal blood flow and, consequently, decreases uric acid clearance.

However, recent animal studies demonstrated that diuretics can prevent hypertension in experimental induced hyperuricemia, but do not block the development of renal arteriolopathy [42, 43]. These studies suggest that diuretic use may diminish the renal blood flow and accelerate the development of renal vascular disease by stimulating the renin-angiotensin system, thus, predisposing the patient to the progression of renal disease. Results of a survey on the changes in drug use patterns of anti-hypertension treatments in the United States suggest that population-wide diuretic use may increase the incidence of end stage renal disease [44]. In clinical trials, the usage of diuretics in the EWPHE [45], Syst-Eur [46], SHEP [47] and INSIGHT [48] studies were all statistically associated with a greater decline in renal function, mainly assessed by a rise in serum creatinine, compared to the other treatment groups. Borgres et al. [49] studied 385 hypertensive women, and showed that hyperuricemia was associated with an increase in inflammatory markers only in patients on diuretic therapy. In a binary logistic regression, hyperuricemia (uric acid >6.0 mg/ dL) was independently associated with chronic kidney disease (eGFR <60 mL/ min / 1.73 m) (OR 2.63, 95% CI 1.61-4.3; P<.001). In hypertensive women, they concluded that the presence of hyperuricemia indicated a substantial degree of kidney dysfunction as well as a greater cardiovascular risk profile. Nevertheless, the study of Lin and colleagues [33] analyzed 2,145 anti-hypertension treated subjects, of those 438 patients were receiving diuretics and 53% had hyperuricemia. The close relationship between serum uric acid and serum creatinine was confirmed by the results of the multiple logistic regression analysis. In the diuretic user group, the higher serum uric acid quartiles were associated with a higher risk of elevated serum creatinine for men (P=0.057 for trend) and women (P=0.0001 for trend). Further linear regression analysis was forced to determine the relationships between serum creatinine, diuretic use, and serum uric acid; and found that there was an insignificant effect of diuretic use on serum creatinine elevation (0.07 mg/dL) in comparison to non-diuretic users. They claim that there is no significant harm associated with diuretic use, and suggest that it is not diuretics that influences serum creatinine, but whether or not they result in serum uric acid elevation. Study results still remain controversial regarding the role of diuretic treatment in renal failure progression. Further clinical placebo control trials are required to evaluate this issue.

Summary

In summary, it is known that there is no single essential cause of cardiovascular renal disease. Uric acid is strongly correlated with hypertension development and cardiovascular renal disease. Renal function impairment may be caused by high blood pressure, diabetes, and dyslipidemia. It remains unclear whether serum uric acid is causally linked to other risk factors for cardiovascular renal disease. However, measuring serum uric acid is a useful test for clinicians as it carries important renal prognostic information, especially in hypertensive patients.

Diuretics effectively lower blood pressure and may be beneficial in hypertensive patients due to end-organ protection. However, diuretics are also associated with elevations of serum uric acid and serum creatinine, and whether they have an adverse effect remains uncertain.

References

[1] Breckenridge A. Hypertension and hyperuricaemia. *Lancet* 1966; 1:15-8.

[2] Hoieggen A, Alderman MH, Kjeldsen SE, et al. The impact of serum uric acid on cardiovascular outcomes in the LIFE study. *Kidney Int.* 2004; 65:1041-9.

[3] Verdecchia P, Schillaci G, Reboldi G, Santeusanio F, Porcellati C, Brunetti P. Relation between serum uric acid and risk of cardiovascular disease in essential hypertension. The PIUMA study. *Hypertension* 2000; 36:1072-8

[4] Franse LV, Pahor M, Di Bari M, et al. Serum uric acid, diuretic treatment and risk of cardiovascular events in the Systolic Hypertension in the Elderly Program (SHEP). *J Hypertens* 2000; 18:1149-54.

[5] Alderman MH, Cohen H, Madhavan S. Distribution and determinants of cardiovascular events during 20 years of successful antihypertensive treatment. *J Hypertens* 1998; 16:761-9.

[6] Bickel C, Rupprecht HJ, Blankenberg S, et al. Serum uric acid as an independent predictor of mortality in patients with angiographically proven coronary artery disease. *Am J Cardiol.* 2002; 89:12-7.

[7] Lee JE, Kim YG, Choi YH, Huh W, Kim DJ, Oh HY. Serum uric acid associated with microalbuminuria in prehypertension. *Hypertension* 2006; 47:96 -67.

[8] Iwashima Y, Horio T, Kamide K, Rakugi H, Ogihara T, Kawano Y. Uric acid, left ventricular mass index, and risk of cardiovascular disease in essential hypertension. *Hypertension* 2006; 47:195-202.

[9] Anker SD, Doehner W, Rauchhaus M, et al. Uric acid and survival in chronic heart failure: validation and application in metabolic, functional, and hemodynamic staging. *Circulation* 2003; 107:1991-7.

[10] Lehto S, Niskanen L, Ronnemaa T, Laakso M. Serum uric acid is a strong predictor of stroke in patients with non-insulin-dependent diabetes mellitus. *Stroke* 1998; 29:635-9.

[11] Culleton BF, Larson MG, Kannel WB, Levy D. Serum uric acid and risk for cardiovascular disease and death: the Framingham Heart Study. *Ann Intern Med.* 1999; 131:7-13.

[12] Fang J, Alderman MH. Serum uric acid and cardiovascular mortality the NHANES I epidemiologic follow-up study, 1971-1992.National Health and Nutrition Examination Survey. *JAMA* 2000; 283:2404-10.

[13] Viazzi F, Parodi D, Leoncini G, et al. Serum uric acid and target organ damage in primary hypertension. *Hypertension* 2005;45:991-6

[14] Alderman MH, Cohen H, Madhavan S, Kivlighn S. Serum uric acid and cardiovascular events in successfully treated hypertensive patients. *Hypertension*. 1999;34:144-50

[15] Kim SY, Guevara JP, Kim KM, Choi HK, Heitjan DF, Albert DA. Hyperuricemia and Risk of Stroke: A systematic review and metaanalysis. *Arthritis Rheum*. 2009; 61: 885–92

[16] Sundstrom J, Sullivan L, D'Agostino RB, Levy D, Kannel WB, Vasan RS. Relations of serum uric acid to longitudinal blood pressure tracking and hypertension incidence. *Hypertension* 2005;45:28-33

[17] Lin CS , Lee WL , Hung YJ , et al. Prevalence of hyperuricemia and its association with antihypertensive treatment in hypertensive patients in Taiwan. *Int J Cardiol* (2010 E pub. ahead of print), doi:10.1016/j.ijcard.2010.10.0

[18] Freedman DS, Williamson DF, Gunter EW, Byers T. Relation of serum uric acid to mortality and ischemic heart disease: the NHANES I epidemiologic follow-up study. *Am J Epidemiol* 1995; 141:637– 44.

[19] Chang HY, Pan WH, Yeh WT, et al. Hyperuricemia and gout in Taiwan: results from the Nutritional and Health Survey in Taiwan (1993–96*). J Rheumatol* 2001; 28: 1640–6.

[20] Selby JV, Friedman GD, Quesenberry CP, Jr. Precursors of essential hypertension: pulmonary function, heart rate, uric acid, serum cholesterol, and other serum chemistries. *Am J Epidemiol.* 1990; 131:1017-27.

[21] Krishnan E, C. Kwoh K, H. Schumacher R, Kuller L. Hyperuricemia and incidence of hypertension among men without metabolic syndrome. *Hypertension*. 2007; 49:298-303

[22] Niskanen LK, Laaksonen DE, NyyssÖnen K, et al. Uric acid level as a risk factor for cardiovascular and all-cause mortality in middle-aged men a prospective cohort study. *Arch Intern Med.* 2004;164:1546-51

[23] Cannon PJ, Stason WB, Demartini FE, Sommers SC, Laragh JH. Hyperuricemia in primary and renal hypertension. *N Engl J Med* 1966; 275:457-64.

[24] Messerli FH, Frohlich ED, Dreslinski GR, Suarez DH, Aristimuno GG. Serum uric acid in essential hypertension: an indicator of renal vascular involvement. *Ann Intern Med* 1980; 93:817-21

[25] Mazzali M, Hughes J, Kim YG, et al. Elevated uric acid increases blood pressure in 398 rat by a novel crystal-independent mechanism. *Hypertension* 2001; 38:1101–6.

[26] Siu YP, Leung KT, Tong MKH, Kwan TH. Use of allopurinol in slowing the progression of renal disease through its ability to lower serum uric acid level. *Am J Kidney Dis* 2005; 47:51-59.

[27] Feig DI, Soletsky B, Johnson RJ. Effect of allopurinol on the blood pressure of adolescents with newly diagnosed essential hypertension. *JAMA* 2008; 300:924–32.

[28] Steele TH. Urate secretion in man: the pyrazinamide suppression test. *Ann Intern Med* 1973; 79:734-7.

[29] Hsu CY, Iribarren C, McCulloch CE, Darbinian J, Go AS. Risk factors for end-stage renal disease: 25-year follow-up. *Arch Intern Med* 2009; 169:342–50.

[30] Obermayr RP, Temml C, Gutjahr G, Knechtelsdorfer M, Oberbauer R, Klauser-Braun R. Elevated uric acid increases the risk for kidney disease. *J Am Soc Nephrol* 2008; 19:2407–13

[31] Iseki K, Oshiro S, Tozawa M, Iseki C, Ikemiya Y, Takishita S. Significance of hyperuricemia on the early detection of renal failure in a cohort of screened subjects. *Hypertens Res* 2001; 24:691–7.

[32] See LC, Kuo CF, Chuang FH, et al. Serum uric acid is independently associated with metabolic syndrome in subjects with and without a low estimated glomerular filtration rate. *J Rheumatol.* 2010; April 22 [E pub. ahead of print].

[33] Lin CS, Hung YJ, Chen GY, et al. A multicenter study of the association of serum uric acid, serum creatinine, and diuretic use in hypertensive patients. *Int J Cardiol* 2011; 148: 325–330

[34] Chonchol M, Shlipak MG, Katz R, et al. Relationship of uric acid with progression of kidney disease. *Am J Kidney Dis* 2007; 50:239-47.

[35] Ben-Dov I Z, Kark JD. Serum uric acid is a GFR-independent long-term predictor of acute and chronic renal insufficiency: the Jerusalem Lipid Research Clinic cohort study. *Nephrol Dial Transplant* 2011 [E pub. ahead of print] 0: 1–9 doi: 10.1093/ndt/gfq740

[36] Iseki K, Oshiro S, Tozawa M, Iseki C, Ikemiya Y, Takishita S. Significance of hyperuricemia as a risk factor for developing ESRD in a screened cohort of screened subjects. *Am J Kidney Dis* 2004; 44:642–50.

[37] Madero M, Sarnak MJ, Wang X, et al. Uric acid and long-term outcomes in CKD. *Am J Kidney Dis* 2009; 53:796–803.

[38] Kanbay M, Ozkara A, Selcoki Y, et al. Effect of treatment of hyperuricemia with allopurinol on blood pressure, creatinine clearence, and proteinuria in patients with normal renal functions. *Int Urol Nephrol* 2007; 39:1227–33

[39] Siu YP, Leung KT, Tong MK, Kwan TH. Use of allopurinol in slowing the progression of renal disease through its ability to lower serum uric acid level. *Am J Kidney Dis* 2006; 47:51–9

[40] George J, Struthers AD. Role of urate, xanthine oxidase and the effects of allopurinol in vascular oxidative stress. *Vascular Health and Risk Management* 2009; 5: 265–72.

[41] Hare JM, Mangal B, Brown J, et al. Impact of oxypurinol in patients with symptomatic heart failure results of the OPT-CHF Study. *J Am Coll Cardiol* 2008; 51:2301–9.

[42] Mazzali M, Kanellis J, Han L, et al. Hyperuricemia induces a primary renal arteriolopathy in rats by a blood pressure-independent mechanism. *Am J Physiol Renal Physiol* 2002; 282:F991–7.

[43] Ono Y, Ono H, Frohlich ED. Hydrochlorothiazide exacerbates nitric oxide-blockade nephrosclerosis with glomerular hypertension in spontaneously hypertensive rats. *J Hypertens* 1996; 14:823–8.

[44] Hawkins RG, Houston MC. Is population-wide diuretic use directly associated with the incidence of end-stage renal disease in the United States? A hypothesis. *Am J Hypertens* 2005; 18:744-9.

[45] Fletcher A, Amery A, Birkenhager W, et al. Risks and benefits in the trial of the European Working Party on High Blood Pressure in the Elderly. *J Hypertens* 1991; 9:225-30

[46] Voyaki SM, Staessen JA, Thijs L, et al. Systolic Hypertension in Europe (Syst-Eur) Trial Investigators. Follow-up of renal function in treated and untreated older patients with isolated systolic hypertension. *J Hypertens* 2001; 19:511–19

[47] Savage PJ, Pressel SL, Curb JD, et al. Influence of long-term low-dose diuretic-based antihypertensive therapy on glucose, lipid, uric acid and potassium levels in older men and women with isolated systolic hypertension. The Systolic Hypertension in the Elderly Program. *Arch Intern Med* 1999; 158:741–751.

[48] Brown MJ, Palmer CR, Castaigne A, et al. Morbidity and mortality in patients randomized to doubleblind treatment with a long-acting calcium-channel blocker or diuretic in the International Nifedipine GITS study: Intervention as a Goal in Hypertension Treatment (INSIGHT). *Lancet* 2000; 356:366–72

[49] Borges RL, Hirota AH, Quinto BM, Ribeiro AB, Zanella MT, Batista MC. Uric acid as a marker for renal dysfunction in hypertensive women on diuretic and nondiuretic therapy. *J Clin Hypertens* 2009, 11::253-9

[50] Kahn HA, Medalie JH, Neufeld HN et al.: The incidence of hypertension and associated factors: The Israel ischemic heart disease study. *Am Heart J,* 1972; 84: 171–82

[51] Hunt SC, Stephenson SH, Hopkins PN, Williams RR. Predictors of an increased risk of future hypertension in Utah: a screening analysis. *Hypertension* 1991; 17:969–76.

[52] Jossa F, Farinaro E, Panico S, et al. Serum uric acid and hypertension: the Olivetti Heart Study. *J Hum Hypertens* 1994; 8:677–81.

[53] Taniguchi Y, Hayashi T, Tsumura K, Endo G, Fujii S, Okada K. Serum uric acid and the risk for hypertension and Type 2 diabetes in Japanese men: the Osaka Health Survey. *J Hypertens* 2001; 19:1209–15.

[54] Masuo K, Kawaguchi H, Mikami H, Ogihara T, Tuck ML. Serum uric acid and plasma norepinephrine concentrations predict subsequent weight gain and blood pressure elevation. *Hypertension* 2003; 42:474–80.

[55] Nakanishi N, Okamoto M, Yoshida H, Matsuo Y, Suzuki K, Tatara K. Serum uric acid and risk for development of hypertension and impaired fasting glucose or Type II diabetes in Japanese male office workers. *Eur J Epidemiol,* 2003; 18: 523–30

[56] Alper AB Jr, Chen W, Yau L, Srinivasan SR, Berenson GS, Hamm LL. Childhood uric acid predicts adult blood pressure: the Bogalusa Heart Study. *Hypertension* 2005; 45:34–8.

[57] Perlstein TS, Gumieniak O, Williams GH, et al. Uric acid and the development of hypertension: the Normative Aging Study. *Hypertension* 2006; 48:1031–6.

[58] Mellen PB, Bleyer AJ, Erlinger TP, et al. Serum uric acid predicts incident hypertension in a biethnic cohort: the Atherosclerosis Risk in Communities study. *Hypertension* 2006; 48:1037–42.

[59] Shankar A, Klein R, Klein BE, Nieto FJ. The association between serum uric acid level and long term incidence of hypertension: population-based cohort study. *J Hum Hypertens* 2006; 20:937–45

[60] Forman JP, Choi H, Curhan GC. Plasma uric acid level and risk for incident hypertension among men. *J Am Soc Nephrol* 2007; 18:287–92..

[61] Krishnan E, Kwoh CK, Schumacher HR, Kuller L. Hyperuricemia and incidence of hypertension among men without metabolic syndrome. *Hypertension* 2007; 49:298–303

[62] Forman JP, Choi H, Curhan GC: Uric acid and insulin sensitivity and risk of incident hypertension. *Arch Intern Med,* 2009; 169:155–62

[63] Zhang W, Sun K, Yang Y, Zhang H, Hu FB, Hui R. Plasma uric acid and hypertension in a chinese community: prospective study and metaanalysis *Clinical Chemistry* 2009; 55:11 2026–34 .

[64] Daoussis D, Panoulas V, Toms T, et al. Uric acid is a strong independent predictor of renal dysfunction in patients with rheumatoid arthritis. *Arthritis Research and Therapy* 2009; 11:R116 (doi:10.1186/ar2775).

[65] Hovind P, Rossing P, Tarnow L, Johnson RJ, Parving HH. Serum uric acid as a predictor for development of diabetic nephropathy in type 1 diabetes an inception cohort study. *Diabetes* 2009; 58:1668–1671,

[66] Weiner DE, Tighiouart H, Elsayed EF, Griffith JL, Salem DN, Levey AS. Uric acid and incident kidney disease in the community. *J Am Soc Nephrol* 2008;19:1204–11.

[67] Chen N, Wang W, Huang Y, et al. Community based study on CKD subjects and the associated risk factors. *Nephrol Dial Transplant* 2009; 24:2117– 23.

[68] Chen YC, Su CT, Wang ST, Lee HD, Lin SY. A preliminary investigation of the association between serum uric acid and impaired renal function. *Chang Gung Med J* 2009; 32:66–71.

[69] Park JT, Kim DK, Chang TI, et al. Uric acid is associated with the rate of residual renal function decline in peritoneal dialysis patients. *Nephrol Dial Transplant* 2009; 24: 3520–3525 .

[70] Sturm G, Kollerits B, Neyer U, Ritz E, Kronenberg F. Uric acid as a risk factor for progression of non-diabetic chronic kidney disease? The Mild to Moderate Kidney Disease (MMKD) Study. *Exp Gerontol* 2008; 43:347–52.

[71] Nakahama K, Inoue T, Iseki K, et al. Hyperuricemia as a predictor of hypertension in a screened cohort in Okinawa, Japan. *Hypertens Res* 2004; 27:835–41.

In: Uric Acid
Editors: S. Castillo and E. Maldonado
ISBN 978-1-62100-762-3

Chapter V

Uric Acid: Biology, Functions and Diseases

Carlos G. Musso, Matilde Navarro, and Manuel Vilas
Nephrology Division, Hospital Italiano de Buenos Aires, Argentina

Abstract

Uric acid is the end-product of the purine metabolism in human beings. Most of this substance is in the form of monosodium urate in compartments with pH 7.4 , such as plasma and extracellular fluids. In urine, where pH can be between 4.7 and 8.0, the ratio of uric acid - urate varies with pH, being this substance entirely as uric acid at acid urine: pH of 5.0 or less. Normal plasma uric acid level is 2.2–7.5 mg/dl in adult males, and it is slightly lower in premenopausal females: 2.1- 6.6 mg/dl. Normally, two-thirds of uric acid is eliminated by the kidney and one-third by the gut. Only 4 % of this substance is bound to plasma proteins, thus most of it is freely filterable and it can be dialyzed from plasma. Around 10 % of the filtrated urate is finally excreted in the urine. In the kidney, uric acid is mainly handled in the proximal tubule where it suffers two processes: reabsorption and secretion. In chronic renal disease serum urate increases at the same rate as creatinine, as creatininemia increases further the uricemia does not, because of an increase in its fractional excretion which can reach 85 % or more in advanced renal failure. Furthermore, there is an increased gut secretion of this substance in this setting. Regarding serum uric acid alterations: Hypouricemia is observed in the setting of uricosuric agents (benzbromarone), proximal tubular dysfunction, and syndrome of inappropriate antidiuretic hormone secretion, hematological malignant disorders and secondary to some drugs such as: corticosteroids, losartan, and low dose of non steroidal anti- inflammatories. Hyperuricemia is observed in gout inflammatory arthritis, acid uric urolithyasis, chronic renal disease, acute hyperuricemic nephropathy (tumoral lysis), and rhabdomyolysis. In conclusion, uric acid comes from purine metabolism, it is mainly excreted by the kidney and its serum levels can be altered by different conditions such as metabolic factors, drug influence, renal disease, and/or tissue destruction.

Keywords: uric acid, metabolism, physiology

Introduction

Uric acid is the end-product of the purine metabolism in human beings, and this substance is synthesized from the xanthine and hypoxanthine bases by the action of the enzyme xanthine oxidoreductase. Since uric acid pK is 5.4, most of it (99%) is in the form of monosodium urate in compartments with pH 7.4 such as plasma and extracellular fluids. In urine, where pH can be between 4.7 and 8.0, the ratio of uric acid - urate varies with pH, being this substance entirely as uric acid at a urine pH of 5.0 or less [1,2].

Uric Acid Metabolism

Normal plasma uric acid level is 2.2–7.5 mg/dl in adult males, and it is slightly lower (2.1- 6.6 mg/dl) in premenopausal females [3]. Normally, two-thirds of uric acid is eliminated by the kidney and one-third by the gut [4]. Only 4 % of this substance is bound to plasma proteins, thus most of it is freely filterable [5]. Around 10 % of the filtrated urate is finally excreted in the urine, being this process usually greater in men in comparison with the female: fractional excretion of uric acid (FEUAc) is around 12% and 8% respectively [2].

In healthy old people, serum uric acid level and FEUAc do not differ compared to the ones in the healthy young population, even though hyper-uricemia is often found in elderly people, mainly in males, perhaps due to the influence of some drugs, such as diuretics [6, 7]. Besides, when healthy old people undergo volume expansion, they show no significant difference between their renal uric excretion before and after the procedure [8].

In the kidney, uric acid is mainly handled in the proximal tubule where it suffers two processes: reabsorption and secretion. Regarding the former, it takes place more specifically in the S_1 segment, being its transport across the brush-border indirectly coupled to sodium transport. On the other hand, uric acid tubular secretion, which takes place in the S_2 segment, appears to be mediated principally by a voltage-sensitive transporter [9,10].

Uric Acid Disorders

Many substances can influence the renal handling of uric acid. Among the ones that reduce its renal excretion we can mention: low doses of cyclo-oxygenase inhibitors, diuretics, pyrazinamide, ethambutol, ethanol and lead intoxication. Conversely, high doses of cyclo-oxygenase inhibitors increase its renal excretion [2,11,12,13].

Hypouricemia may be observed in the setting of uricosuric agents (benzbromarone, probenecid), allopurinol (xanthine oxidase inhibition), acquired proximal tubular defects (Fanconi syndrome) such as Wilson disease, syndrome of inappropriate antidiuretic hormone secretion, haematological malignant disorders and as a consequence of using some drugs such as: corticosteroids, losartan, and low dose of non steroidal anti- inflammatories [2, 12, 13, 15, 16, 17].

Hyperuricemia may be observed in gout inflammatory arthritis, acid uric urolithyasis, toxemia of pregnancy, polycythemia vera, response to treatment of pernicious anemia (peak precedes maximum reticulocyte count by about 24 hours), chronic renal disease, cytotoxic drugs: acute hyperuricemic nephropathy (tumoral lysis), lead poisoning (plumbism), sarcoidosis, lactic acidosis, hypo-thyroidism, dysparathyroidism, alcoholism, cirrhosis, rhabdomyolysis (crush injuries, prolonged immobilization), severe psoriasis, storage diseases (von Gierke´s disease) [12,13,18,19,20].

The uric acid-creatinine ratio has been proposed: serum uric acid (mg/dl) / serum creatinine (mg/dl) as marker for distinguishing an acute renal failure due to hyperuricemia (ratio > 1.0) from one secondary to other mechanism [13].

In the majority of patients with gout, hyperuricaemia results from a poly-genically inherited tendency to a reduced fractional excretion of uric acid, coupled almost always with a large intake of dietary purine. In this context, there is increased uric acid tubular reabsorption since FEUAc is around 5% [18].

Even though at the beginning of chronic renal disease serum urate increases at the same rate as the creatinine does, as the creatininemia increases further the uricemia does not, because of an increase in its fractional excretion which can reach 85 % or more in advanced renal failure. Furthermore, there is an increased gut secretion of this substance in this setting [19].

Additionally, it has been documented that increased serum uric acid levels are strongly associated with prevalent chronic kidney disease, increased frequency and risk of gout episode, and with higher total and gout-related direct healthcare cost per episode, higher risk of mortality in hemodialysis patients (J-shaped association), and an independent risk factor for cardio-vascular disease in high-risk individuals [21,22;23,24].

Conclusion

Uric acid comes from purine metabolism, it is mainly excreted by the kidney and its serum levels can be altered by different conditions such as metabolic factors, drug influence, renal disease, and/or tissue destruction.

References

[1] Stone TW, Simmonds HA. Purines: *Basic and clinical aspects.* London. Kluwer. 1991.

[2] Beck L. Transtornos clinicos del metabolismo del ácido úrico. In Beck L (Ed). Clinicas medicas de Norteamérica. Mexico. Iteramericana. 1981: 397-408.

[3] Hershfield M. Gout and uric acid metabolism. In Bennett JC, Plum F (Eds). *Cecil Textbook of Medicine.* Philadelphia. WB Saunders Company. 1996: 1508-1515.

[4] Sorensen LB. Gout secondary to chronic renal disease: studies on urate metabolism. *Annals of rheumatic diseases.* 1980, 39: 424-430.

[5] Kovarsky J, Holmes E, Kelley WN. Absence of significant urate binding to plasma proteins. *Journal of laboratory and clinical medicine.* 1979, 93: 85-91.

[6] Lai S, Tan C, Ng K. Epidemiology of hyperuricemia in the elderly. *Yale Journal of Biology and Medicine*. 2001; 74:151-157.

[7] Takala J, Anttila S, Gref C, Isomaki H. *Scand J Rheumatology*. 1988; 17: 155-160.

[8] Musso CG, Alvarez Gregory J, Macías Núñez JF. Renal handling of uric acid, magnesium, phosphorus, calcium, and acid base in the elderly. In Macías Núñez, Cameron S, Oreopoulos D (Eds). *Renal Ageing : Health and Disease. 2008*: 155-171.

[9] Maesaka JK, Fishbane S. Regulation of renal urate excretion: a critical review. *American Journal of Kidney Diseases.* 1998, 32: 917-933.

[10] Grassl SM. Facilitated diffusion of urate in avian brush border membrane vesicles. *American Journal of physiology, cell physiology.* 2002, 283: c1155-c1162.

[11] Cameron S, Simmonds A. *Uric Acid.* In Cameron S (Ed). Oxford. Oxford Textbook of Nephrology. 2006.

[12] Caspi D, Lubart E, Graff E, Habot B, Yaron M, Segal R. The effect of mini-dose aspirin on renal function and uric acid handling in the elderly patients. *Arthritis and Rheumatism.* 2000; 43: 103-108.

[13] Gomella L. *Manual de referencia para el médico.* Buenos Aires. Panamericana. 1990.

[14] Wallach J. *Interpretation of diagnostic tests.* Boston. Little, Brown and Company.1992.

[15] Keidar S, Kohan R, Levy J, Grenadier E, Palant A, Ben-Ari J. Non-oliguric acute renal failure alter treatment with sulfinpyrazone. *Clinical nephrology.* 1982, 17: 266-267.

[16] Sommers DK, Shoenman HS. Drug interactions with urate excretion in man. *European journal of pharmacology.* 1987, 32: 499-502.

[17] Bunier M, Roch-Ramel F, Brunner HR. Renal effects of angiotensin II receptor blockade in normotensive subjects. *Kidney International.* 1996. 49, 1787-1790.

[18] Rodríguez Mañas L, Solís Jiménez J. *Patología reumatológica en geriatría.* In Salgado A, Guillén F, Ruipérez I (Eds). Barcelona. Masson. 2002: 477-492.

[19] Danovitch GM, Weinberger J, Berlyne GM. Uric acid in advanced renal failure. *Clinical Science.* 1972,43: 331-341.

[20] Jones DP, Mahmoud H, Chesney RW. Tumor lysis syndrome: pathogenesis and management. *Pediatric Nephrology.* 1995, 9: 206-212.

[21] Chonchol M, Shlipak M, Katz R, Sarnak M, Newman A, Siscovick D, Kestenbaum B, Carney J, Fried L. Relationship of uric acid with

progression of kidney disease. *American Journal of Kidney Diseases.* 2007; 50(2): 239-247.

[22] Wu E, Patel P, Mody R, Yu A, Cahill K, Tang J, Krishnan E. Frequency, risk, and cost of gout-related episodes among the elderly: does serum uric acid level matter? *The Journal of Rheumatology*. 2009; 36: 1032-1040.

[23] Hsu S, Pai M, Peng Y, Chiang C, Ho T, Hung K. Serum uric acid levels show a "J-shaped" association with all-cause mortality in haemodialysis patients. *Nephrol Dial Transplant.* 2004. 19: 457- 462.

[24] Baker J, Krishnan E, Chen L, Schumacher R. Serum uric and cardiovascular disease: recent developments, and where do they leave us? *The American Journal of Medicine*. 2005; 118: 816-826.

In: Uric Acid
Editors: S. Castillo and E. Maldonado
ISBN 978-1-62100-762-3

Chapter VI

Uric Acid, Urea and Creatinine: Implications for Patients with Diabetic Vascular Disease*

Hairong Nan†
The Hong Kong Institute of Diabetes and Obesity,
The Chinese University of Hong Kong, Hong Kong SAR, China

Abstract

This chapter deals with the positive association between serum UA and cardiovascular disease, which has been found not only in the high risk factor population but also in the general population. We summarize the association of UA within the literature and the underlying mechanisms of UA with cardiovascular disease in diabetic patients, starting with the antioxidant prooxidant UA redox shuttle, followed by the association between UA and inflammation. We also discuss prognostic implications of uric acid, urea and creatinin in diabetic patients, with cautionary notes about their clinical management.

---

*Versions of these chapters were also published in *Diabeto-Angiology,* edited by Marijan Bosevski, published by Nova Science Publishers, Inc. They were submitted for appropriate modifications in an effort to encourage wider dissemination of research.

†E-mail: jh_nan@cuhk.edu.hk

Keywords: Uric acid, Urea, Creatinine, Cardiovascular disease, Cardio-metabolic risk factors, Diabetes

Introduction

The positive association between serum UA, coronary artery disease and cardiovascular diseases has been recognized for 50 years [1, 2.] The issue of elevated serum UA or hyperuricemia as an independent risk factor for atherosclerotic cardiovascular disease (CVD) has received much renewed interest in recent years. Many reviews and editorials provide different views [3-6] and some studies provide conflicting results [7-10]. Johnson et al. [11] have summarized that hyperuricemia predicted the development of CVD, not only in individuals with hypertension or preexisting CVD but also in the general population. Whereas, Wheeler et al. [12] considered that measurement of serum UA levels is unlikely to usefully enhance the prediction of coronary heart disease or to be a major determinant of the disease in the general populations based on the results of a meta-analysis of data of 15 prospective studies. Although some studies suggested that serum UA is an independent risk factor for coronary artery disease [1, 9, 10, 13]. There is still more evidence that the association of hyperuricaemia with coronary artery disease events is dependent on the association between serum UA and other risk factors, such as hypertension, obesity and elevated levels of triglycerides [7, 8, 13-15]. This evidence suggest that the influence of UA on coronary artery disease is explained by the secondary association of UA with other established etiological risk factors (hypertension, dyslipidaemia, hyperinsulinaemia, obesity and pre-existing disease) [16]. Studies on the influence of urea and creatinine on the prognosis of patients with diabetic vascular disease have been mentioned, previously. Overall, a causal role for hyperuricemia in CVD events and mortality has not been unequivocally established [11]. Serum UA may, however, provide useful prognostic information in subjects with diabetes and vascular complications.

1. UA Associated with Cardio-Metabolic Risk Factors

The clustering of resistance to insulin-stimulated glucose uptake, hyper-insulinemia, hyperglycemia, hyperuricemia, increased very low-density lipoprotein, triglycerides, decreased high-density lipoprotein cholesterol (HDL-C), and hypertension has been noticed and described since 1923 [17] named later as "syndrome X" [18], "Insulin resistance (IR) syndrome" [19] or more recently the "metabolic syndrome" [20]. The co-morbidities associated with hyperuricemia include obesity, hyperlipidemia, hypertension, IR, hyperglycemia, CVD (coronary artery disease and stroke), and chronic renal disease [11].

1.1. Obesity

Obesity has reached epidemic proportions in the past decade and possibly represents the most important cardio-metabolic factor. The association of hyperuricemia with obesity has been recognized for hundreds of years [21]. Hyperuricemia has been associated with increasing body mass index (BMI) in early studies. A high correlation between serum UA, weight and body surface area was found in American Indians in 1966 [22], in the same year a similar association between serum UA and body size was discovered in the European population [23] and in a population of the Marian Island as well [24]. The concept of central obesity was first introduced by Vague in the1940s [25], later on, in1956 he pointed out for the first time that central obesity (android) was more important than peripheral obesity (gynaecoid) in relation to diabetes, atherosclerosis, gout and urate calculus diseases.

Recent follow-up studies further clarify the picture of the relationship between serum UA and obesity. A few epidemiology studies have shown that BMI is definitely the strongest positive factor correlating with serum UA among components of cardio-metabolic risk factors including hypertension, high triglycerides, fatty liver and lower HDL-C in all sex-race groups after adjustment for possible confounders including age, education, physical activity, smoking, alcohol intake, oral contraceptive use and creatinine [9, 26; 27].

Obesity has several effects on UA metabolism, including increased UA production and decreased renal UA clearance [28]. In obese subjects, hyperuricemia is attributable to the overproduction of UA and impairment in the renal clearance of UA, owing to the influence of hyperinsulinemia secondary to IR [29-31]. Weight reduction is associated with moderate calorie and carbohydrate restriction and increased proportional intake of protein and unsaturated fat (as recommended for insulin-resistant states) is reported to be accompanied by a decrease in serum UA levels and dyslipidemia in gout patients [32].

Similarly, the amelioration of IR by either a low-energy diet or troglitazone decreased the serum UA levels in overweight hypertensive individuals [33].

A possible role of leptin in the relationship among hyperuricemia, obesity and IR has been addressed recently. Leptin, a hormone product of the obese gene, is expressed in adipocytes and acts through the hypothalamus to regulate food intake and energy expenditure. Most obese people show leptin resistance, and increased leptin levels are significantly associated with IR among non-diabetic individuals [34]. Insulin responses, triglyceride levels and BMI are independently and significantly associated with leptin concentrations [35]. A body of studies among healthy male adolescents [36], obese children [37], and in moderately obese women [38] imply that the association of serum UA, obesity and IR may, at least in part, be mediated by leptin expression 39].

1.2. Dyslipidemia

An association between hypertriglyceridemia and hyperuricemia is well established [40]: up to 80% of individuals with hypertriglyceridemia have hyperuricemia, and 50% to 75% of gouty patients have hypertriglyceridemia; obesity and excessive alcohol intake may be confounders of the relations between hypertriglyceridemia and hyperuricemia. However, it is not suspected that dyslipidaemia, especially hypertriglyceridamia, is involved and interacting in association with serum UA with obesity, irrespective of central or peripheral type of obesity.

More recently, free fatty acids have been discovered as being related to hyperuricemia independently of hypertriglyceridemia, obesity and central body fat distribution [41, 42]. Elevated serum total cholesterol and triglyceride concentrations were observed among patients in the highest percentile of serum UA levels compared with those in the lowest percentile, and an inverse relationship was seen between HDL-C and serum UA levels [43].

Concentrations of serum lipoprotein Lp(a), apolipoproteins A-II, B, C-II, C-III and E were also reported as being increased, while HDL–C decreased in patients with gout [44]. The prevalence of the apolipoprotein E2 allele was greater in gout patients, and its presence was associated with higher tri-glyceride levels in very low-density lipoprotein and intermediate-density lipo-proteins, and with reduced renal UA excretion [45]. A corollary of these observations is that individuals with both hyperuricemia and hyperlipidemia, particularly those with abdominal obesity, may be at high-risk for type 2 diabetes and CVDs.

1.3. Hypertension

The relationship of UA to hypertension is independent of obesity, renal function or anti-hypertensive medications, especially thiazide diuretics [46]. This association has been well demonstrated in many clinical and epidemiological studies [9, 42, 47]. Hyperuricemia is common in patients with essential hypertension. It appears that overall about 25% of hypertensive individuals have hyperuricaemia, and this figure increases to 75% in those with malignant hypertension [11, 48]. Studies suggested that hyperuricemia in hypertensive subjects reflected early renal vascular involvement associated with hypertension [49, 50]. Several studies, however, found that elevated serum UA appeared in hypertension patients without clinical renal dysfunction.

Univariate associations of hyperuricaemia with both systolic and diastolic BP were attenuated after adjustment for BMI, suggesting a major role of adiposity in this association [8, 16].

Furthermore, results from most population-based epidemiological studies have approved that hyperuricemia is a significant independent predictor for incident hypertension by higher relative risk in Korean [51], Italian [52], Canadian [53], American black from the US [54, 55], native Japanese [56] and Japanese immigrants in the US [57].

New findings from a number of animal model experimental studies shed light on a causal role for hyperuricemia in hypertension [58-60[. This strongly suggests that both angiotensin II and nitric oxide are involved in the pathogenesis of the hypertension induced by UA.

The underlying mechanisms of increases in the UA level with essential hypertension are still not well understood. Recent studies proposed the role of IR being the possible pathophysiological link between an altered tubular sodium handling and UA metabolism in humans [26, 50, 61-63].

1.4. Insulin Resistance

The Bruneck Study, based on a random sample of the general population (n = 888, aged 40-79), reported that the prevalence of IR is 62.8% in subjects with hyperuricemia [64]. IR is probably one of the underlying conditions triggering the development of the above metabolic disorders.

The increased purine biosynthesis and turnover, with consequent increases in serum UA concentrations caused by the increased activity of the hexose monophosphate shunt, may be linked to IR and/or hyperinsulinemia [65]. Especially, the impairment of the glycolytic pathway can increase the flux of glucose-6-phosphate through the hexose monophosphate shunt, resulting in the accumulation of ribose-5-phosphate and other intermediates, which are major substrates for UA production [66, 67]. On the other hand, there is evidence that UA may not only be a consequence of IR, but it may actually promote or worsen IR. Moreover, a recent study [68] showed that UA plays an important role in the pathogenesis of metabolic syndrome, probably due to its ability to inhibit endothelial function by inhibiting nitric oxide bioavailability [69]. Since insulin needs nitric oxide to stimulate glucose uptake, the investigators hypothesized that hyperuricemia may have a key role in the pathogenesis of IR [68].

Furthermore, insulin receptors were found in different tubular segments of the kidney in humans [70]. Insulin can enhance renal proximal tubular UA reabsorption in humans due to an active transport mechanism closely linked to the tubular reabsorption of sodium [31, 63, 71].

Whatever the site of the tubular effects of insulin, the possible mechanisms linking hyperinsulinemia (a consequence of IR) with hyperuricemia include the direct stimulations of tubular ion (UA-Na) exchange or the acceleration of cellular metabolism [72]. In addition, drugs that improve insulin sensitivity, such as metformin [73], troglitazone [33], sibutramine [74, 75], and orlistat [73, 76] can also lower UA levels.

1.5. UA and Its Changes with Pre-Diabetes and Type 2 Diabetes

A few cross-sectional studies have also shown that diabetic patients have the lowest levels of all UA levels [77-79]; the UA concentration was significantly elevated in people with IGT [79], IFG and newly diagnosed diabetes in white populations [80, 81]. A study among Chinese in Taiwan [82] revealed that among non-diabetic subjects, FPG increased with increasing UA levels in women, but not in men. Our investigation in the Chinese population in northern mainland China further confirmed previous findings, despite the differences in assays used for the UA and in diagnostic criteria for diabetes in different studies [83].

Very few studies have investigated the relationship between 2hPG and UA due to the fact that 2h OGTT have not been widely applied. A population-based cross-sectional study revealed that serum UA was strongly correlated with 2hPG in non-diabetic Mauritian men (r=0.15) and women (r=0.22) ($p<0.001$ for both) [84].

We found in a previous study a weak UA-2hPG association in the year 2002 [83]. In our 2006 study the UA-2hPG association seemed stronger in men than in women, while the UA-FPG association was stronger in women than in men {Nan, 2009 #1109}. Since the cross-sectional studies were confounded by many concurrent conditions, the prospective implications of the UA levels in diagnosing diabetes need to be further investigated.

Age, BMI, triglycerides, creatinine, C-reactive protein, blood pressure or treatment for hypertension, and alcohol intake for men, particularly, fasting insulin in higher ranges of plasma glucose distribution, are the important confounding factors for the association of serum UA with FPG and 2hPG. It probably reflected the biochemical interaction between glucose, insulin and purine metabolism, with increased excretions of UA during hyperglycaemia and glycosuria [65, 71, 81].

UA Predicts Incident Type 2 Diabetes

To our knowledge, only a few studies have investigated the relationship between fasting serum UA and type 2 diabetes incidences, and most of these studies were conducted in the male population alone [85-90]. Similar to these previous studies, recently, a population-based longitudinal study over a maximum of 11 years of follow-up in Mauritian [91], and another community-based prospective cohort study of 2,690 Chinese participants (age range, 35-97 years) over a median follow-up of 9.0 years in Chin-Shan town, Taiwan [92] have found that high baseline UA levels predicted future type 2 diabetes development.

In the 13-year follow up of the Rancho Bernardo study of 566 older middle class Caucasians, each 1 mg/dl increment in UA level independently predicted incident type 2 diabetes among participants who had impaired fasting glucose (odds ratio 1.75, 95% CI 1.1-2.9, $P = 0.02$) [90]. The baseline serum UA level has also been found to independently predict the 2-hPG levels during 13.5 years of follow-ups in a Swedish male population, with a low regression coefficient of 0.01 ($p=0.026$) [93].

In the Finnish Diabetes Prevention Study [94] in high-risk middle-aged subjects with IGT, baseline UA and its changes predicted a 2-fold increase in the likelihood of developing type 2 diabetes. Furthermore, UA and its changes during follow-up were related to corresponding changes in FPG and 2-hPG [94].

2. Underlying Mechanisms of UA with CVD in Diabetes Patients [95]

2.1. Antioxidant – Prooxidant UA Redox Shuttle

The term "Oxidative Stress" was generally denoted as "the disturbance in prooxidant-antioxidant balance in favor of the former" in 1985 by Helmut Sies [96]. The interest for elucidating the molecular mechanisms underlying the effects of oxidative stress on cells has been greatly increased during the past few years, mainly due to proposals indicating its involvement in many physiological and pathological conditions, including ageing, cancer and atheriosclerosis [97]. It should be noted that low levels of reactive oxygen species are continuously present in cells under physiological conditions, and the cellular redox state is tightly regulated. The toxic effects of reactive oxygen species become apparent only when the rate of their generation increases and the defence capacity of cells are overwhelmed. Oxidative stress has been regarded broadly as a mediator in the process of development of CVD [98, 99]. Oxidative stress may also play a role in the pathogenesis of diabetes, associated cardiac dysfunction, general vascular dysfunction and the metabolic syndrome [100, 101].

Serum UA in the early stages of the atherosclerotic process is known to act as an antioxidant and may be one of the strongest contents of plasma antioxidative capacity [97, 102]. The simple concept is intriguing that serum UA in patients with CVD, the metabolic syndrome, type 2 diabetes, hypertension, and renal disease may reflect a compensatory mechanism to counter oxidative stress. However, this is not able to explain why higher serum UA levels in patients with these diseases are generally associated with worse outcomes [11].

Unfortunately, later in the atherosclerotic process when serum UA levels are above the normal range 357 μmol/l in females and 387–416 μmol/l in males, the previously antioxidant (UA) paradoxically becomes prooxidant [9, 103]. This antioxidant – prooxidant UA redox shuttle (Figure 1) seems to depend strongly on its surrounding environment such as timing (early or late in the disease process), location of the tissue and substrate, acidity (acidic–, basic– or neutral PH value), the surrounding oxidant milieu, the depletion of other local antioxidants, the supply and duration of oxidant substrate and its oxidant enzyme. Depletion of local antioxidants with an underlying increase in oxidantive -redox stress is associated with the uncoupling of the endothelial nitric oxide synthase enzyme, then a decrease in the locally produced naturally occurring antioxidants, endothelial nitric oxide and endothelial dysfunction [104]. This process is also occurring within the microvascular bed at the level of the capillary within various affected hypertensive and diabetic end organs [104-106].

Recent experimental studies [102, 105-107] have explored the formation of UA being connected with the conversion of xanthine dehydrogenase to xanthine oxidase, which leads to concomitant production of free radicals. Glantzounis et al. reviewed [97] that beyond the well-known reasons for an increase in the serum UA level there stands another poorly recognized factor, i.e. local ischemia, from the metabolism of hypoxanthine-xanthine by the enzyme xanthine oxidoreductase. In this respect, it is worth noting that xanthine oxidoreductase occurs in two different forms. Xanthine dehydrogenase is the prevalent operative form under physiological conditions and has a greater affinity for oxidized nicotinamide adenine dinucleotide compared with oxygen, as the electron acceptor. Under ischemic conditions, in parallel to the degradation of ATP into adenine and an extensive conversion of xanthine dehydrogenase to xanthine oxidase takes place. The latter utilizes molecular oxygen in place of oxidized nicotinamide adenine dinucleotide as an electron acceptor, leading to the formation of superoxide anion and hydrogen peroxide, which in parallel with UA production [97].

2.2. Serum UA and Inflammation

Increased serum UA was closely associated with systemic inflammation, such as elevated C-reactive protein (CRP) [108], stimulation of release of chemokine monocyte chemoattractant protein-1[109], interleukin-6 and tumor necrosis factor-α synthesis [110]. Serum UA has been shown to have a significant positive correlation with CRP in Japanese men (n=3,692) aged 34–69 years [111], in a German population-based study (n=1,703, aged 18-89 years) [112], and in a representative random sample of 957 individuals aged 65-95 years of the Italian general population [113]. In the Italian study [113], the association between UA and CRP was independent of multiple confounders of white blood cells, neutrophil count, interleukin-6, interleukin-1 receptor antagonist, interleukin-18, and tumor necrosis factor-α. The relationship of UA with inflammatory markers is linear across the entire range of UA levels.

Moreover, a follow-up study [114] in the same Italian cohort found that (1) baseline UA and changes in UA from baseline to follow-up were significant predictors of CRP changes during a 3-year follow-up, independent of baseline inflammatory markers and relevant confounders; (2) subjects in the fourth and fifth UA quintiles had a higher probability of developing clinically relevant increased interleukin-6 (>2.5 pg/ml) and CRP (>3 mg/l) during the 3-year follow-up period, compared with those in the second quintile. A clinical study of a sample of 30 patients concluded that serum UA may reflect the severity of systolic dysfunction and the activation of inflammation in patients with congestive heart failure [115].

Serum UA elevation may indeed be a sensitive marker for underlying vascular inflammation and remodeling within the arterial vessel wall and capillary interstitium. Some evidence suggests that UA may exert a negative effect on CVD by stimulating inflammation, which is clearly involved in the pathogenesis of CVD [116, 117]. Is it possible that serum UA levels could be as similarly predictive as CRP since it is a sensitive marker for underlying inflammation and remodeling within the arterial vessel wall and the myocardium? It is not surprising that these two markers of risk track together within the metabolic syndrome and CVD [104].

In spite of the evidence that UA might contribute to the development of human vascular disease and atherosclerosis through a pro-inflammatory pathway, the relationship between UA and inflammation has been less investigated and need further exploration.

Moreover, since UA has been demonstrated to independently correlate with arterial stiffness and hsCRP, however, hsCRP was not correlated with arterial stiffness. Authors speculated that the association of UA with increased cardiovascular risks in hypertension was probably contributed by both increased arterial stiffness and enhanced inflammation [118].

2.3. Endothelial Dysfunction

Vascular endothelial dysfunction involves a very early stage of vascular disease, which may occur at any level in the arterial system. It contributes to the development and progression of atherosclerosis by favoring coagulation, cell adhesion and inflammation by promoting inappropriate vasoconstriction and/or vasodilation, and by enhancing transendothelial transport of atherogenice lipoproteins [119].

Since one of the major sites of the production of UA in the cardiovascular system is the vessel wall, particularly the endothelium [120] and UA's ability to inhibit endothelial function through inhibiting nitric oxide bioavailability

[69], elevated serum UA may be a marker of endothelial dysfunction. It has been shown that UA concentrations correlated inversely with flow-mediated brachial artery vasodilation in vivo [121].

Moreover, in a controlled setting of dietary treatment with an arginine-enriched nutrient bar, which enhances nitric oxide activity, the increased flow mediated dilation was associated with the reduction of UA levels [121].

In summary, experimental evidence suggests a complex but potentially direct causal relationship between serum UA and numerous deleterious biologic functions which are involved in the pathogenesis of metabolic syndrome and atherosclerosis [122-125].

Table 1. Possible roles of hyperuricemia in the metabolic syndrome and cardiovascular diseases [95]

Components	Potential mechanisms
Hypertension	1. Urate reabsorption increased in settings of increased renal vascular resistance, microvascular disease predisposed to tissue ischemia that leads to increased urate generation (excess purine metabolism) and reduced excretion (due to lactate competing with urate transporter in the proximal tubule) 2. Increased oxidative – redox stress 3. Antioxidant – Prooxidant Paradox:Urate Redox Shuttle 4. UA effect on the renin-angiotensin system.
Obesity – Insulin resistance	1. Overproduction of UA and impairment in renal clearance of UA 2. Leptin may induce hyperuricemia. 3. Insulin increases sodium reabsorption and is tightly linked to urate reabsorption.
Glucose intolerance and/or Diabetes	Acting through obesity and insulin resistance.
Dyslipidaemia	Link between fatty acid synthesis and production of NADPH.
Accelerated atherosclerosis	1. Endothelial dysfunction 2. Accelerated atherosclerosis with increased vascular cell apoptosis 3. Inflammatory necrosis with increased purine metabolism resulting in hyperuricemia 4. Increased oxidative stress through ischemia-reperfusion and xanthine oxidase 5. Antioxidant – Prooxidant Paradox: Urate Redox Shuttle 6. UA effect on the renin-angiotensin system.

For example, in vitro studies showed that UA stimulates both vascular smooth muscle cell proliferation and the release of chemotactic and inflammatory substances [122, 125, 126], induces monocyte chemotaxis [127], inhibits endothelial cell proliferation and migration [128, 129], and causes oxidative stress in adipocytes, which results in impaired secretion of adiponectin [130]. The role of serum UA in the development of metabolic abnormalities is summarized in Table 1 according to current understanding.

3. Prognostic Implications of Serum Creatinine, Urea and Uric Acid in Diabetic Patients

A serum creatinine with a concentration greater than 1.5 mg/dl has been reported as a strong predictor of CVD in patients in the Hypertension Detection and Follow-up Program (HDFP) [131]. In the HDFP study, a linear positive association was found between serum creatinine concentration and cardiovascular mortality over the 5-year follow up, with a 5-fold difference between the lowest and the highest strata (serum creatinine < 1.5 *v.s* > 1.7 mg/dl).

Mann et al. have carried out a random clinical trail, based on the Heart Outcomes and Prevention Evaluation (HOPE) study [132], among 980 patients with mild renal insufficiency (serum creatinine concentration >/=1.4 mg/dl) and 8,307 patients with normal renal function (serum creatinine concentration <1.4 mg/dl). They indicated that mild renal insufficiency is a new risk factor for future cardiovascular events in patients with other risk factors for CVD. The risk associated with mild renal insufficiency was substantial and was independent of other known risk factors, such as hypertension, diabetes, and microalbuminuria. Increased serum creatinine concentration and microalbuminuria were equally strong renal-related risk predictors but were independent of each other. Moreover, the effect of increased serum creatinine concentration was as strong in non-diabetic patients as in those with diabetes. This concerns the fact that about one third of the patients with renal insufficiency have microalbuminuria, and detecting both biological markers may benefit intervention treatment early.

Unpublished data of the editor Dr. Bosevski included 370 pts with type 2 diabetes and coronary artery disease enrolled in a cross sectional study. Multiple linear regression analysis was built to define the factors of peripheral arterial disease measured by ABI value. Regression analysis defined the mean and minimal values of ABI to be associated independently with diabetes duration (β 0,120, Sig 0,025) and blood urea level (β -0,126, Sig 0,019).

Previous studies reported that ABI value was associated with arterial hypertension, albuminuria and blood creatinin level in the diabetic population.[132a,b] These results have clinical implications in defining pts with higher diabetes duration and blood urea level with a greater probability for detection of pathological ankle-brachial index.

The Framingham study was the first to examine the independent association between serum UA level elevation and cardiovascular outcomes in the general population, but it failed to provide consistent conclusions in 2 separate investigations [7, 133]. Nevertheless in another national-wide survey, the NHANES I study, of 5,926 subjects followed for an average of 16.4 years, the increasing serum UA concentration was related to increasing cardiovascular mortality in both sexes and ethnic groups [9]. Death due to ischemic heart disease and overall cardiovascular mortality rates increased in relation to UA quartiles (relative risk, 1.77 in men and 3.00 in women), even after adjustment for age, race, BMI, smoking, alcohol intake, cholesterol, hypertension, and diabetes. Recently, a study of 1,017 patients with angiographically proven coronary artery disease has shown a 5-fold increase in overall mortality rates among patients with serum UA levels in the top quartile, compared with those in the lowest quartile. In addition, serum UA was an independent predictor of mortality in patients with coronary artery disease after adjustment for 12 variables (including diuretic use) that influence overall cardiovascular mortality [134]. In patients with well-controlled hypertension, cardiovascular mortality was significantly greater among hyperuricemic individuals than among their normouricemic counterparts [135].

More recently, elevated serum UA has been shown as being an independent predictor of mortality in high-risk groups including subjects with hypertension, coronary heart disease [136], stroke [137], and heart failure [138]. A similar result was further confirmed in a population-based cohort study of 12-years follow-ups in middle-aged healthy Finnish men. The predictive value of hyperuricemia with respect to cardiovascular outcome is not weakened by adjustment for the components of metabolic syndrome, including fasting insulin levels [103]. A study in apparently healthy Japanese men revealed a significant and positive relationship between high serum UA and electrocardiographically-diagnosed left ventricular hypertrophy (ECG-LVH) [139]. The association was independent of age, degree of obesity, renal function, hypertension and other potential confounding factors, including diabetes, and also revealed a significant independent association to hypertensive subjects.

Currently, however, a paucity of studies have explored the association between serum UA levels and CVD outcome in the type 2 diabetic population. In a cohort study [140] involving 2,726 type 2 diabetic outpatients, who were followed for a mean period of 4.7 years, the elevated serum UA, corresponding to one SD increase, had 1.3 increased odds of cardiovascular death after multivariable adjustment.

Whereas the association of serum UA with all-cause mortality did not. The authors concluded that higher serum UA levels are associated with increased risk of CVD mortality in type 2 diabetic individuals, independent of conventional risk factors, such as adiposity, smoking, hypertension, dyslipidemia, diabetes duration, glycemic control, medication use, and renal function measures.

A prospective comprehensive 8.2 year follow up study was carried out in 41,879 men and 48,514 women ages >35 years in the general population from Taiwan. It demonstrated that hyperuricemia is an independent risk factor for all-cause and cardiovascular mortality in the Taiwanese general population, in high-risk groups (patients with hypertension and diabetes), and potentially in low-risk groups (those with low metabolic risk, such as triglycerides <150 mg/dl, glucose <100 mg/dl, BMI <27 kg/m^2, systolic blood pressure <130 mm Hg, diastolic blood pressure <85 mm Hg, and with no history of receiving medications for blood pressure or diabetes). The adjusted risks increased 8–13% with every mg/dl increase of serum UA level for all-cause and cardiovascular mortality. The hazard ratio for cardiovascular mortality was 1.6 in diabetic patients [141]. Although, whether increased serum UA concentrations are just a risk indicator or a causative risk factor of CVD cannot be determined from such epidemiological studies.

A systemic review has recently summarized relevant studies concerning UA and possible links to hypertension, renal disease, and CVD in a very comprehensive way [142].

Right now there is not sufficient data to support the general treatment of asymptomatic hyperuricemia to reduce cardiovascular risk, although such evidence is mounting. However, there would seem to be a body of evidence to warrant clinical trials to determine whether lowering UA levels would be of clinical benefit in the prevention or treatment of cardiovascular and renal diseases [142].

Conclusion

Plasma creatinin determination is useful for the prognosis of patients with diabetic vascular disease. The prognostic value of UA and urea in the development of type 2 diabetes is not clear, and the direction of causality between hyperuricemia and metabolic risk factors is uncertain. Further studies to investigate the pathophysiological mechanism underlying the relationship between glucose and UA, and between cardio-metabolic risk factors and UA, may help to understand the formation of these metabolic disorders and find a way to stop or delay the development of diabetes and CVDs.

Regardless of the pathophysiological explanations, these observations raise an important clinical question. Is it possible to prevent/postpone the onset of type 2 diabetes by reducing serum UA in people with pre-diabetes? Recently, in a short-term, crossover designed clinical trial of adolescents with newly diagnosed hypertension, treatment with allopurinol resulted in a reduction of blood pressure [143]. The results represent a new potential therapeutic approach, although not a fully developed therapeutic strategy due to potential adverse effects. These preliminary findings require confirmation in larger randomized, controlled clinical trails. Allopurinol and other agents of febuxostat, or pegylated, would be potential candidate drugs for intervention, but the safety and cost-effectiveness of these medications in pre-diabetes or diabetes first need to be studied.

Reference

[1] Gertler M, Garn S, Levine S. Serum uric acid in relation to age and physique in health and coronary heart disease. *Ann. Intern. Med.* 1951;34:1421-1431.

[2] Klein R, Klein B, Cornoni J, Maready J, Cassel J, Tyroler H. Serum uric acid: Its relationship to coronary heart disease risk factors and cardiovascular disease, Evans County, Georgia. *Arch. Intern. Med.* 1973;132:401-410.

[3] Dobson A. Is raised serum uric acid a cause of cardiovascular disease or death? *Lancet.* Nov 6 1999;354(9190):1578.

[4] Johnson RJ, Kivlighn SD, Kim YG, Suga S, Fogo AB. Reappraisal of the pathogenesis and consequences of hyperuricemia in hypertension,

cardiovascular disease and renal disease. *Am. J. Kidney Dis.* 1999;33:225-234.

[5] Yusuf S, Bosch J. Urate levels as a predictor of cardiac deaths: causal relation or mere association? *Eur. Heart J.* May. 2002;23(10):760-761.

[6] Alderman M, Aiyer KJ. Uric acid: role in cardiovascular disease and effects of losartan. *Curr. Med. Res. Opin.* 2004;20(3):369-379.

[7] Culleton BF, Larson MG, Kannel WB, Levy D. Serum uric acid and risk for cardiovascular disease and death: the Framingham Heart Study. *Ann. Intern. Med.* Jul 6 1999;131(1):7-13.

[8] Wannamethee SG, Shaper AG, Whincup PH. Serum urate and the risk of major coronary heart disease events. *Heart.* Aug 1997;78(2):147-153.

[9] Fang J, Alderman MH. Serum uric acid and cardiovascular mortality the NHANES I epidemiologic follow-up study, 1971-1992. National Health and Nutrition Examination Survey. *JAMA.* 2000;283(18):2404-2410.

[10] Liese A, Hense H, Lowel H, Doring A, Tietze M, Keil U. Association of serum uric acid with all-cause and cardiovascular disease mortality and incident myocardial infarction in the MONICA Augsburg cohort. *Epidemiology.* 1999;10:391-397.

[11] Johnson RJ, Kang DH, Feig D, et al. Is there a pathogenetic role for uric acid in hypertension and cardiovascular and renal disease? *Hypertension.* Jun 2003;41(6):1183-1190.

[12] Wheeler JG, Juzwishin KD, Eiriksdottir G, Gudnason V, Danesh J. Serum uric acid and coronary heart disease in 9,458 incident cases and 155,084 controls: prospective study and meta-analysis. *PLoS Med.* Mar 2005;2(3):e76.

[13] Freedman D, Williamson D, Gunter E, Byers T. Relation of serum uric acid to mortality and ischemic heart disease. The NHANES I epidemiologic follow-up study. *Am. J. Epidemiol.* 1995;141:637-644.

[14] Jee SH, Lee SY, Kim MT. Serum uric acid and risk of death from cancer, cardiovascular disease or all causes in men. *Eur. J. Cardiovasc. Prev. Rehabil.* Jun 2004;11(3):185-191.

[15] Yano K, Reed DM, McGee DL. Ten-year incidence of coronary heart disease in the Honolulu Heart Program. Relationship to biologic and lifestyle characteristics. *Am. J. Epidemiol.* May 1984;119(5):653-666.

[16] Wannamethee SG. Serum Uric Acid and Risk of Coronary Heart Disease. *Curr. Pharm Des.* 2005;11(32):4125-4132.

[17] Kylin E. Studies of the hypertension-hyperglycemia hyperuricemia syndrome (Studien ueber das hypertonie-hypergly-kämie-

hyperurikämiesyndrom.). *Zentral-blatt fuer Innere Medizin.* 1923;44:105-127.

[18] Reaven GM. Banting lecture 1988. Role of insulin resistance in human disease. *Diabetes.* December 1, 1988 1988;37(12):1595-1607.

[19] Haffner S, Valdez R, Hazuda H, Mitchell B, Morales P, Stern M. Prospective analysis of the insulin-resistance syndrome (syndrome X). *Diabetes.* June 1, 1992 1992;41(6):715-722.

[20] Grundy SM. Hypertriglyceridemia, insulin resistance, and the metabolic syndrome. *Am J Cardiol.* May 13 1999;83(9B):25F-29F.

[21] Wynagaarden J, Kelley W. Gout. In: Stanbury J, Wynagaarden J, Fredrickson D, Goldstein J, Brown M, eds. *The Metabolic Basis of Inherited Disease.* New York: McGraw-Hill; 1983:1043-1114.

[22] O'Brien WM, Burch TA, Bunim JJ. Genetics of hyperuricaemia in Blackfeet and Pima Indians. *Ann Rheum Dis.* Mar 1966;25(2):117-119.

[23] Krizek V. Serum uric acid in relation to body weight. *Ann. Rheum. Dis.* Sep 1966;25(5):456-458.

[24] Burch TA, O'Brien WM, Need R, Kurland LT. Hyperuricaemia and gout in the Mariana Islands. *Ann. Rheum. Dis.* Mar 1966;25(2):114-116.

[25] Vague J. La differenciation sexuelle. Facteur determinant des formes de l'obesite. *Press Med.* 1947;30:339-340.

[26] Rathmann W, Funkhouser E, Dyer AR, Roseman JM. Relations of hyperuricemia with the various components of the insulin resistance syndrome in young black and white adults: the CARDIA study. Coronary Artery Risk Development in Young Adults. *Ann. Epidemiol.* 1998;8(4):250-261.

[27] Ogura T, Matsuura K, Matsumoto Y, et al. Recent trends of hyperuricemia and obesity in Japanese male adolescents, 1991 through 2002. *Metabolism.* 2004;53(4):448-453.

[28] Emmerson BT. Alteration of urate metabolism by weight reduction. *Aust. NZJ Med.* Aug 1973;3(4):410-412.

[29] Yamashita S, Matsuzawa Y, Tokunaga K, Fujioka S, Tarui S. Studies on the impaired metabolism of uric acid in obese subjects: marked reduction of renal urate excretion and its improvement by a low-calorie diet. *Int. J. Obes.* 1986;10(4):255-264.

[30] Matsuura F, Yamashita S, Nakamura T, et al. Effect of visceral fat accumulation on uric acid metabolism in male obese subjects: visceral fat obesity is linked more closely to overproduction of uric acid than subcutaneous fat obesity. *Metabolism.* 1998;47(8):929-933.

[31] Quinones Galvan A, Natali A, Baldi S, et al. Effect of insulin on uric acid excretion in humans. *Am. J. Physiol.* 1995;268(1 Pt 1):E1-5.

[32] Dessein PH, Shipton EA, Stanwix AE, Joffe BI, Ramokgadi J. Beneficial effects of weight loss associated with moderate calorie/carbohydrate restriction, and increased proportional intake of protein and unsaturated fat on serum urate and lipoprotein levels in gout: a pilot study. *Ann. Rheum. Dis.* Jul 2000;59(7):539-543.

[33] Tsunoda S, Kamide K, Minami J, Kawano Y. Decreases in serum uric acid by amelioration of insulin resistance in overweight hypertensive patients: effect of a low-energy diet and an insulin-sensitizing agent. *Am. J. Hypertens.* Aug 2002;15(8):697-701.

[34] Donahue RP, Prineas RJ, Donahue RD, et al. Is fasting leptin associated with insulin resistance among nondiabetic individuals? The Miami Community Health Study. *Diabetes Care.* Jul 1999;22(7):1092-1096.

[35] Ruige JB, Dekker JM, Blum WF, et al. Leptin and variables of body adiposity, energy balance, and insulin resistance in a population-based study. The Hoorn Study. *Diabetes Care.* Jul 1999;22(7):1097-1104.

[36] Ogura T, Matsuura K, Otsuka F, et al. Serum leptin correlates with serum uric acid but not serum testosterone in non-obese male adolescents. *Res. Commun. Mol. Pathol. Pharmacol.* 2000;107(1-2):55-64.

[37] Moreno LA, Pineda I, Rodriguez G, et al. Leptin and metabolic syndrome in obese and non-obese children. *Horm. Metab. Res.* Jul 2002;34(7):394-399.

[38] Garcia-Lorda P, Bullo M, Vila R, del Mar Grasa M, Alemany M, Salas-Salvado J. Leptin concentrations do not correlate with fat mass nor with metabolic risk factors in morbidly obese females. *Diabetes Nutr. Metab.* Dec 2001;14(6):329-336.

[39] Bedir A, Topbas M, Tanyeri F, Alvur M, Arik N. Leptin might be a regulator of serum uric acid concentrations in humans. *Jpn. Heart J.* 2003;44(4):527-536.

[40] Barlow KA. *Hyperlipidemia in primary gout. 0026-0495.* Mar 1968;17(3):289-299.

[41] Bonora E, Targher G, Zenere M, et al. Relationship of uric acid concentration to cardiovascular risk factors in young men. The role of obesity and central fat distribution. The Verona Young Men Atherosclerosis Risk Factors Study. *Int. J. Obes. Relat. Metab. Disord.* 1996;20:975-980.

[42] Conen D, Wietlisbach V, Bovet P, et al. *Prevalence of hyperuricemia and relation of serum uric acid with cardiovascular risk factors in a developing country. 1471-2458.* 2004;4(1):9.

[43] Matsubara M, Chiba H, Maruoka S, Katayose S. Elevated serum leptin concentrations in women with hyperuricemia. *J. Atheroscler. Thromb.* 2002;9(1):28-34.

[44] Takahashi S, Yamamoto T, Moriwaki Y, Tsutsumi Z, Higashino K. Increased concentrations of serum Lp(a) lipoprotein in patients with primary gout. *Ann. Rheum. Dis.* Feb 1995;54(2):90-93.

[45] Cardona F, Tinahones FJ, Collantes E, Escudero A, Garcia-Fuentes E, Soriguer FJ. The elevated prevalence of apolipoprotein E2 in patients with gout is associated with reduced renal excretion of urates. *Rheumatology (Oxford).* Mar 2003;42(3):468-472.

[46] Heinig M, Johnson RJ. Role of uric acid in hypertension, renal disease, and metabolic syndrome. *Cleve. Clin. J. Med.* Dec 2006;73(12):1059-1064.

[47] Li Y, Stamler J, Xiao Z, Folsom A, Tao S, Zhang H. Serum uric acid and its correlate in Chinese adult population, urban and rural, of Beijing. The PRC-USA Collaborative Study in Cardiovascular and Cardiopulmonary Epidemiology. *Int. J. Epidemiol.* 1997;26(2):288-296.

[48] Cannon P, Stason W, Demartini F, Sommers S, Laragh J. Hyperuricemia in primary and renal hypertension. *N. Engl. J. Med.* 1966;275:457-464.

[49] Messerli F, Froehlich E, Dreslinski G, Suarez D, Aristimuno G. Serum uric acid in essential hypertension: an indicator of renal vascular involvement. *Ann. Intern. Med.* 1980;93:817-821.

[50] Frohlich ED. Uric acid. A risk factor for coronary heart disease. *JAMA.* Jul 21 1993;270(3):378-379.

[51] Yoo TW, Sung KC, Shin HS, et al. Relationship between serum uric acid concentration and insulin resistance and metabolic syndrome. *Circulation Journal.* Aug 2005;69(8):928-933.

[52] Jossa F, Farinaro E, Panico S, et al. Serum uric acid and hypertension: the Olivetti heart study. *J. Hum. Hypertens.* 1994;8(9):677-681.

[53] Forman JP, Choi H, Curhan GC. Plasma uric acid level and risk for incident hypertension among men. *J. Am. Soc. Nephrol.* Jan 2007;18(1):287-292.

[54] Dyer AR, Liu K, Walsh M, Kiefe C, Jacobs DR, Jr., Bild DE. Ten-year incidence of elevated blood pressure and its predictors: the CARDIA study. Coronary Artery Risk Development in (Young) Adults. *J. Hum. Hypertens.* Jan 1999;13(1):13-21.

[55] Mellen PB, Bleyer AJ, Erlinger TP, et al. Serum uric acid predicts incident hypertension in a biethnic cohort: the atherosclerosis risk in communities study. *Hypertension.* Dec 2006;48(6):1037-1042.

[56] Nagahama K, Inoue T, Iseki K, et al. Hyperuricemia as a predictor of hypertension in a screened cohort in Okinawa, Japan. *Hypertens Res.* Nov 2004;27(11):835-841.

[57] 5Imazu M, Yamamoto H, Toyofuku M, et al. Hyperinsulinemia for the development of hypertension: data from the Hawaii-Los Angeles-Hiroshima Study. *Hypertens Res.* Sep 2001;24(5):531-536.

[58] Sanchez-Lozada LG, Tapia E, Santamaria J, et al. Mild hyperuricemia induces vasoconstriction and maintains glomerular hypertension in normal and remnant kidney rats. *Kidney Int.* 2005;67(1):237-247.

[59] Nakagawa T, Mazzali M, Kang DH, et al. Hyperuricemia causes glomerular hypertrophy in the rat. *Am. J. Nephrol.* 2003;23(1):2-7.

[60] Sanchez-Lozada LG, Nakagawa T, Kang DH, et al. Hormonal and cytokine effects of uric acid. *Curr. Opin. Nephrol. Hypertens.* Jan 2006;15(1):30-33.

[61] Facchini F, Chen YD, Hollenbeck CB, Reaven GM. Relationship between resistance to insulin-mediated glucose uptake, urinary uric acid clearance, and plasma uric acid concentration. *JAMA.* Dec 4 1991;266(21):3008-3011.

[62] Lee J, Sparrow D, Vokonas P, Landsberg L, Weiss S. Uric acid and coronary heart disease risk: evidence for a role of uric acid in the obesity-insulin resistance syndrome. *Am. J. Epidemiol.* 1995;142(3):288-294.

[63] Cappuccio FP, Strazzullo P, Farinaro E, Trevisan M. Uric acid metabolism and tubular sodium handling. Results from a population-based study. *JAMA.* Jul 21 1993;270(3):354-359.

[64] Bonora E, Kiechl S, Willeit J, et al. Prevalence of insulin resistance in metabolic disorders: the Bruneck Study. *Diabetes.* 1998;47(10):1643-1649.

[65] Modan M, Halkin H, Karasik A, Lusky A. Elevated serum uric acid--a facet of hyperinsulinaemia. *Diabetologia.* Sep 1987;30(9):713-718.

[66] Fox IH. *Metabolic basis for disorders of purine nucleotide degradation. 0026-0495.* 1981;30(6):616-634.

[67] Fox IH, John D, DeBruyne S, Dwosh I, Marliss EB. *Hyperuricemia and hypertriglyceridemia: metabolic basis for the association. 0026-0495.* Aug 1985;34(8):741-746.

[68] Nakagawa T, Hu H, Zharikov S, et al. A causal role for uric acid in fructose-induced metabolic syndrome. *Am. J. Physiol. Renal. Physiol.* Mar 2006;290(3):625-631.
[69] Baldus S, Koster R, Chumley P, et al. Oxypurinol improves coronary and peripheral endothelial function in patients with coronary artery disease. *Free Radic. Biol. Med.* Nov 1 2005;39(9):1184-1190.
[70] Nakamura R, Emmanouel DS, Katz AI. Insulin binding sites in various segments of the rabbit nephron. *J. Clin. Invest.* Jul 1983;72(1):388-392.
[71] Muscelli E, Natali A, Bianchi S, et al. Effect of insulin on renal sodium and uric acid handling in essential hypertension. *Am. J. Hypertens.* 1996;9(8):746-752.
[72] Mandel LJ. Primary active sodium transport, oxygen consumption, and ATP: coupling and regulation. *Kidney Int.* Jan 1986;29(1):3-9.
[73] Gokcel A, Gumurdulu Y, Karakose H, et al. Evaluation of the safety and efficacy of sibutramine, orlistat and metformin in the treatment of obesity. *Diabetes Obes Metab.* Jan 2002;4(1):49-55.
[74] Tambascia MA, Geloneze B, Repetto EM, Geloneze SR, Picolo M, Magro DO. Sibutramine enhances insulin sensitivity ameliorating metabolic parameters in a double-blind, randomized, placebo-controlled trial. *Diabetes Obes Metab.* Sep 2003;5(5):338-344.
[75] Filippatos TD, Kiortsis DN, Liberopoulos EN, Mikhailidis DP, Elisaf MS. A review of the metabolic effects of sibutramine. *Curr. Med Res. Opin.* 2005;21(3):457-468.
[76] Kiortsis DN, Filippatos TD, Elisaf MS. The effects of orlistat on metabolic parameters and other cardiovascular risk factors. *Diabetes Metab.* Feb 2005;31(1):15-22.
[77] Herman JB, Medalie JH, Goldbourt U. Diabetes, prediabetes and uricaemia. *Diabetologia.* 1976;12(1):47-52.
[78] Yano K, Hoads G, Kagan A. Epidemiology of serum urate levels among 8000 Japanese-American men in Hawaii. *J. Chronic. Dis.* 1977;30:171-184.
[79] Tuomilehto J, Zimmet P, Wolf E, Taylor R, Ram P, King H. Plasma uric acid level and its association with diabetes mellitus and some biological parameters in a biracial population of Fiji. *Am. J. Epidemiol.* 1988;127:321-336.
[80] Whitehead TP, Jungner I, Robinson D, Kolar W, Pearl A, Hale A. Serum urate, serum glucose and diabetes. *Ann. Clin. Biochem.* 1992;29(Pt 2):159-161.

[81] Cook DG, Shaper AG, Thelle DS, Whitehead TP. Serum uric acid, serum glucose and diabetes: relationships in a population study. *Postgrad. Med. J.* Nov 1986;62(733):1001-1006.

[82] Chou P, Lin KC, Lin HY, Tsai ST. Gender differences in the relationships of serum uric acid with fasting serum insulin and plasma glucose in patients without diabetes. *J. Rheumatol.* 2001;28(3):571-576.

[83] Nan H, Dong Y, Gao W, Tuomilehto J, Qiao Q. Diabetes associated with a low serum uric acid level in a general Chinese population. *Diabetes Res. Clin. Pract.* Apr 2007;76(1):68-74.

[84] Hodge AM, Boyko EJ, de Courten M, et al. Leptin and other components of the Metabolic Syndrome in Mauritius--a factor analysis. *Int. J. Obes. Relat. Metab. Disord.* 2001;25(1):126-131.

[85] Perry IJ, Wannamethee SG, Walker MK, Thomson AG, Whincup PH, Shaper AG. Prospective study of risk factors for development of non-insulin dependent diabetes in middle aged British men. *BMJ.* Mar 4 1995;310(6979):560-564.

[86] Meisinger C, Thorand B, Schneider A, Stieber J, Doring A, Lowel H. Sex differences in risk factors for incident type 2 diabetes mellitus: the MONICA Augsburg cohort study. *Arch. Intern. Med.* Jan 14 2002;162(1):82-89.

[87] Nakanishi N, Okamoto M, Yoshida H, Matsuo Y, Suzuki K, Tatara K. Serum uric acid and risk for development of hypertension and impaired fasting glucose or Type II diabetes in Japanese male office workers. *Eur J. Epidemiol.* 2003;18(6):523-530.

[88] Lin KC, Tsai ST, Lin HY, Chou P. Different progressions of hyperglycemia and diabetes among hyperuricemic men and women in the kinmen study. *J. Rheumatol.* 2004;31(6):1159-1165.

[89] Dehghan A, van Hoek M, Sijbrands EJ, Hofman A, Witteman JC. High serum uric acid as a novel risk factor for type 2 diabetes. *Diabetes Care.* Feb 2008;31(2):361-362.

[90] Kramer CK, von Muhlen D, Jassal SK, Barrett-Connor E. Serum uric acid levels improve prediction of incident type 2 diabetes in individuals with impaired fasting glucose: the Rancho Bernardo Study. *Diabetes Care.* Jul 2009;32(7):1272-1273.

[91] Nan H, Qiao Q, Soderberg S, et al. Serum uric acid and incident diabetes in Mauritian Indian and Creole populations. *Diabetes Res. Clin. Pract.* May 2008;80(2):321-327.

[92] Chien KL, Chen MF, Hsu HC, et al. Plasma uric acid and the risk of type 2 diabetes in a Chinese community. *Clin. Chem.* Feb 2008;54(2):310-316.

[93] Ohlson LO, Larsson B, Bjorntorp P, et al. Risk factors for type 2 (non-insulin-dependent) diabetes mellitus. Thirteen and one-half years of follow-up of the participants in a study of Swedish men born in 1913. *Diabetologia.* Nov 1988;31(11):798-805.

[94] Niskanen L, Laaksonen DE, Lindstrom J, et al. Serum uric acid as a harbinger of metabolic outcome in subjects with impaired glucose tolerance: the Finnish Diabetes Prevention Study. *Diabetes Care.* Mar 2006;29(3):709-711.

[95] Nan H. *Serum uric acid and metabolic risk factors in three ethnic groups: Asian Indians and Creoles in Mauritius and Chinese in Qingdao, China* [PhD.]. Helsinki: Department of Public Health, University of Helsinki 2008.

[96] Sies H, Cadenas E. Oxidative stress: damage to intact cells and organs. *Philos. Trans. R. Soc. Lond B Biol. Sci.* Dec 17 1985;311(1152):617-631.

[97] Glantzounis GK, Tsimoyiannis EC, Kappas AM, Galaris DA. Uric Acid and Oxidative Stress. *Curr. Pharm. Des.* 2005;11(32):4145-4151.

[98] Berges A, Van Nassauw L, Bosmans J, Timmermans JP, Vrints C. Role of nitric oxide and oxidative stress in ischaemic myocardial injury and preconditioning. *Acta. Cardiol.* Apr 2003;58(2):119-132.

[99] Linke A, Recchia F, Zhang X, Hintze TH. Acute and chronic endothelial dysfunction: implications for the development of heart failure. *Heart Fail Rev.* Jan 2003;8(1):87-97.

[100] Channon KM, Guzik TJ. Mechanisms of superoxide production in human blood vessels: relationship to endothelial dysfunction, clinical and genetic risk factors. *J. Physiol. Pharmacol.* Dec 2002;53(4 Pt 1):515-524.

[101] Deedwania PC. Mechanisms of endothelial dysfunction in the metabolic syndrome. *Curr. Diab. Rep.* Aug 2003;3(4):289-292.

[102] Nyyssonen K, Porkkala-Sarataho E, Kaikkonen J, Salonen J, T. Ascorbate and urate are the strongest determinants of plasma antioxidative capacity and serum lipid resistance to oxidation in Finnish men. *Atherosclerosis.* 1997;130(1-2):223-233.

[103] Niskanen LK, Laaksonen DE, Nyyssonen K, et al. Uric acid level as a risk factor for cardiovascular and all-cause mortality in middle-aged

men: a prospective cohort study. *Arch. Intern. Med.* 2004;164(14):1546-1551.

[104] Hayden MR, Tyagi SC. Uric acid: A new look at an old risk marker for cardiovascular disease, metabolic syndrome, and type 2 diabetes mellitus: The urate redox shuttle. *Nutr. Metab (Lond).* Oct 19 2004;1(1):10.

[105] Bagnati M, Perugini C, Cau C, Bordone R, Albano E, Bellomo G. When and why a water-soluble antioxidant becomes pro-oxidant during copper-induced low-density lipoprotein oxidation: a study using uric acid. *Biochem J.* May 15 1999;340 (Pt 1):143-152.

[106] Patterson RA, Horsley ET, Leake DS. Prooxidant and antioxidant properties of human serum ultrafiltrates toward LDL: important role of uric acid. *J. Lipid. Res.* Mar 2003;44(3):512-521.

[107] Sanguinetti SM, Batthyany C, Trostchansky A, et al. Nitric oxide inhibits prooxidant actions of uric acid during copper-mediated LDL oxidation. *Arch. Biochem. Biophys.* Mar 15 2004;423(2):302-308.

[108] Anker SD, Doehner W, Rauchhaus M, et al. Uric acid and survival in chronic heart failure: validation and application in metabolic, functional, and hemodynamic staging. *Circulation.* Apr 22 2003;107(15):1991-1997.

[109] Kanellis J, Watanabe S, Li JH, et al. Uric acid stimulates monocyte chemoattractant protein-1 production in vascular smooth muscle cells via mitogen-activated protein kinase and cyclooxygenase-2. *Hypertension.* 2003;41(6):1287-1293.

[110] Johnson RJ, Rodriguez-Iturbe B, Kang DH, Feig DI, Herrera-Acosta J. A unifying pathway for essential hypertension. *Am. J. Hypertens.* Mar 2005;18(3):431-440.

[111] Tamakoshi K, Yatsuya H, Kondo T, et al. The metabolic syndrome is associated with elevated circulating C-reactive protein in healthy reference range, a systemic low-grade inflammatory state. *Int. J. Obes Relat Metab Disord.* Apr 2003;27(4):443-449.

[112] Frohlich M, Imhof A, Berg G, et al. Association between C-reactive protein and features of the metabolic syndrome: a population-based study. *Diabetes Care.* Dec 2000;23(12):1835-1839.

[113] Ruggiero C, Cherubini A, Ble A, et al. Uric acid and inflammatory markers. *Eur. Heart J.* May 2006;27(10):1174-1181.

[114] Ruggiero C, Cherubini A, Miller E, 3rd, et al. Usefulness of uric acid to predict changes in C-reactive protein and interleukin-6 in 3-year period

in Italians aged 21 to 98 years. *Am. J. Cardiol.* Jul 1 2007;100(1):115-121.

[115] Olexa P, Olexova M, Gonsorcik J, Tkac I, Kisel'ova J, Olejnikova M. Uric acid--a marker for systemic inflammatory response in patients with congestive heart failure? *Wien Klin. Wochenschr.* Mar 28 2002;114(5-6):211-215.

[116] Hansson GK. Inflammation, atherosclerosis, and coronary artery disease. *N. Engl. J. Med.* Apr 21 2005;352(16):1685-1695.

[117] Festa A, Haffner SM. Inflammation and cardiovascular disease in patients with diabetes: lessons from the Diabetes Control and Complications Trial. *Circulation.* May 17 2005;111(19):2414-2415.

[118] Tsai W-C, Huang Y-Y, Lin C-C, et al. Uric acid is an independent predictor of arterial stiffness in hypertensive patients. *Heart Vessels.* 2009;24(5):371-375.

[119] Aengevaeren WR. Beyond lipids - the role of the endothelium in coronary artery disease. *Atherosclerosis.* Sep 9 1999;147 Suppl 1:S11-16.

[120] Becker BF. Towards the physiological function of uric acid. *Free Radic. Biol. Med.* Jun 1993;14(6):615-631.

[121] Maxwell AJ, Bruinsma KA. Uric acid is closely linked to vascular nitric oxide activity. Evidence for mechanism of association with cardiovascular disease. *J. Am. Coll. Cardiol.* Dec 2001;38(7):1850-1858.

[122] Watanabe S, Kang DH, Feng L, et al. Uric acid, hominoid evolution, and the pathogenesis of salt-sensitivity. *Hypertension.* 2002;40(3):355-360.

[123] Kang DH, Nakagawa T, Feng L, et al. A role for uric acid in the progression of renal disease. *J. Am. Soc. Nephrol.* Dec 2002;13(12):2888-2897.

[124] Mazzali M, Hughes J, Kim YG, et al. Elevated uric acid increases blood pressure in the rat by a novel crystal-independent mechanism. *Hypertension.* Nov 2001;38(5):1101-1106.

[125] Mazzali M, Kanellis J, Han L, et al. Hyperuricemia induces a primary renal arteriolopathy in rats by a blood pressure-independent mechanism. *American Journal of Physiology. Renal Physiology.* 2002;282(6):F991-997.

[126] Rao GN, Corson MA, Berk BC. Uric acid stimulates vascular smooth muscle cell proliferation by increasing platelet-derived growth factor A-chain expression. *J. Biol. Chem.* May 5 1991;266(13):8604-8608.

[127] Zare F, Magnusson M, Bergstrom T, et al. Uric acid, a nucleic acid degradation product, down-regulates dsRNA-triggered arthritis. *J. Leukoc. Biol.* Mar 2006;79(3):482-488.

[128] Kang DH, Park SK, Lee IK, Johnson RJ. Uric acid-induced C-reactive protein expression: implication on cell proliferation and nitric oxide production of human vascular cells. *J. Am. Soc. Nephrol.* Dec 2005;16(12):3553-3562.

[129] Khosla UM, Zharikov S, Finch JL, et al. Hyperuricemia induces endothelial dysfunction. *Kidney Int.* 2005;67(5):1739-1742.

[130] Sautin YY, Nakagawa T, Zharikov S, Johnson RJ. Adverse effects of the classic antioxidant uric acid in adipocytes: NADPH oxidase-mediated oxidative/nitrosative stress. *Am. J. Physiol. Cell Physiol.* Aug 2007;293(2):C584-596.

[131] Shulman NB, Ford CE, Hall WD, et al. Prognostic value of serum creatinine and effect of treatment of hypertension on renal function. Results from the hypertension detection and follow-up program. The Hypertension Detection and Follow-up Program Cooperative Group. *Hypertension.* May 1989;13(5 Suppl):I80-93.

[132] Mann JF, Gerstein HC, Pogue J, Bosch J, Yusuf S. Renal insufficiency as a predictor of cardiovascular outcomes and the impact of ramipril: the HOPE randomized trial. *Ann. Intern. Med.* 2001;134(8):629-636.

[133] Guerrero A, Montes R, Muñoz-Terol J, Gil-Peralta A, Toro J, Naranjo M, et al. Peripheral arterial disease in patients with stages IV and V chronic renal failure. *Nephrol. Dial. Transplant.* 2006 Dec;21(12):3525-31.

[134] O'Hare AM, Rodriguez RA, Bacchetti P. Low ankle-brachial index associated with rise in creatinine level over time: results from the atherosclerosis risk in communities study. *Arch. Intern. Med.* 2005 11;165(13):1481-5.

[135] Abbott RD, Brand FN, Kannel WB, Castelli WP. Gout and coronary heart disease: the Framingham Study. *J. Clin. Epidemiol.* 1988;41(3):237-242.

[136] Bickel C, Rupprecht HJ, Blankenberg S, et al. Serum uric acid as an independent predictor of mortality in patients with angiographically proven coronary artery disease. *Am. J. Cardiol.* Jan 1 2002;89(1):12-17.

[137] Alderman MH, Cohen H, Madhavan S, Kivlighn S. Serum uric acid and cardiovascular events in successfully treated hypertensive patients. *Hypertension.* Jul 1999;34(1):144-150.

[138] Hoieggen A, Alderman MH, Kjeldsen SE, et al. The impact of serum uric acid on cardiovascular outcomes in the LIFE study. *Kidney Int.* 2004;65(3):1041-1049.

[139] Weir CJ, Muir SW, Walters MR, Lees KR. Serum urate as an independent predictor of poor outcome and future vascular events after acute stroke. *Stroke.* 2003;34(8):1951-1956.

[140] Gerber Y, Tanne D, Medalie JH, Goldbourt U. Serum uric acid and long-term mortality from stroke, coronary heart disease and all causes. *Eur. J. Cardiovasc. Prev. Rehabil.* Apr 2006;13(2):193-198.

[141] Mitsuhashi H, Yatsuya H, Matsushita K, et al. Uric Acid and Left Ventricular Hypertrophy in Japanese Men. *Circulation Journal.* 2009;73(4):667-672.

[142] Zoppini G, Targher G, Negri C, et al. Elevated serum uric acid concentrations independently predict cardiovascular mortality in type 2 diabetic patients. *Diabetes Care.* 2009;32(9):1716-1720.

[143] Chen JH, Chuang SY, Chen HJ, Yeh WT, Pan WH. Serum uric acid level as an independent risk factor for all-cause, cardiovascular, and ischemic stroke mortality: a Chinese cohort study. *Arthritis Rheum.* Feb 15 2009;61(2):225-232.

[144] Feig DI, Kang DH, Johnson RJ. Uric acid and cardiovascular risk. *N. Engl. J. Med.* Oct 23 2008;359(17):1811-1821.

[145] Feig DI, Soletsky B, Johnson RJ. Effect of allopurinol on blood pressure of adolescents with newly diagnosed essential hypertension: a randomized trial. *JAMA.* Aug 27 2008;300(8):924-932.

Index

B

C

D

E

M

N

O

P

S

T

U

V

W

Y